Emoji in Higher Education

Emoji are a significant development in contemporary communication, deserving serious attention for their impact on both language use and society. Based on original mixed-methods research, this timely book focuses on emoji literacy across the healthcare landscape, with emphasis on how they are employed in healthcare worker and patient education. It situates emoji within a semioliteracy theoretical framework and presents the findings of a mixed methods study of emoji use as a literacy tool in a health professions course. Drawing on real-life case studies, it explores emoji literacy across a range of public health education contexts including doctor-to-industry, patient-to-doctor, doctor-to-patient, and healthcare providers/CDC to global audience. It also advances a broader argument about the role of emoji in a paradigm shift of communication in education. This title is part of the Flip it Open Programme and may also be available Open Access. Check our website Cambridge Core for details.

OMONPEE W. PETCOFF is Assistant Professor of Reading and Writing at Tarrant County College. Her work promotes semioliterate approaches to teaching literacy skills to struggling adult readers and writers.

JANICE C. PALAGANAS is Professor of Health Professions Education at MGH Institute of Health Professions. She is an award-winning author of textbooks and research articles in team communication and learning.

MARCEL DANESI is Professor Emeritus at the Department of Anthropology, University of Toronto. His notable publications include *The Semiotics of Emoji* (2017) and *Understanding Nonverbal Communication* (2022).

Emoji in Higher Education

A Healthcare-Based Perspective

Omonpee W. Petcoff

Tarrant County College

Janice C. Palaganas

MGH Institute of Health Professions

Marcel Danesi

University of Toronto

CAMBRIDGE
UNIVERSITY PRESS

CAMBRIDGE
UNIVERSITY PRESS

Shaftesbury Road, Cambridge CB2 8EA, United Kingdom

One Liberty Plaza, 20th Floor, New York, NY 10006, USA

477 Williamstown Road, Port Melbourne, VIC 3207, Australia

314–321, 3rd Floor, Plot 3, Splendor Forum, Jasola District Centre, New Delhi – 110025, India

103 Penang Road, #05–06/07, Visioncrest Commercial, Singapore 238467

Cambridge University Press is part of Cambridge University Press & Assessment, a department of the University of Cambridge.

We share the University's mission to contribute to society through the pursuit of education, learning and research at the highest international levels of excellence.

www.cambridge.org
Information on this title: www.cambridge.org/9781009254007

DOI: 10.1017/9781009253994

When citing this work, please include a reference to the DOI 10.1017/9781009253994

First published 2024

A catalogue record for this publication is available from the British Library.

A Cataloging-in-Publication data record for this book is available from the Library of Congress.

ISBN 978-1-009-25400-7 Hardback

Contents

Figures and Tables

Graphic representations of emoji (included in Figures 1.4 and 3.2; in Tables 3.1, 5.2, and 5.2; and on pages 126 and 129) created by graphic artist Elijah Tan

Figures

Tables

Foreword

As a scholar of rhetoric, I have always been intrigued by both verbal and visual systems of communication. For years I taught a seminar on the History of Writing, where we studied the clay "envelopes" containing inscribed tokens used in the ancient Near East and described by Denise Schmandt-Besserat, the cave paintings from Indonesia, France, and Spain, Indigenous rock carvings in the United States, and more elaborate systems such as hieroglyphics. We experimented with setting type on an 1850s Albion press, using handmade paper and marveling at the time about the infinite care it took to set and print even a short poem. We studied ASL and learned about braille. We wrote histories of our own writing, beginning with the first word we remembered inscribing – often a name, impressed into sand or dirt.

Throughout, we puzzled over the relationship between sight and sound, between words and images, and about how such relationships affected our understanding of the world and our ability to communicate within it.

No wonder, then, that when I first began seeing emoji some twenty-five years ago, they already seemed familiar. The ubiquitous smiley face that began popping up in the occasional student note or essay was soon joined by dozens of other images, and while they were ignored by almost all educators and descried as representing marks of illiteracy – or perhaps just bad manners – they proliferated. And they fascinated me.

Today, emoji are an established means of communication, appearing in more and more print and digital publications and gaining attention and interest in fields as diverse as education, government, business, engineering, and healthcare.

Enter O. W. Petcoff, whose use of emoji in her developmental writing classes provided inspiration for her 2023 dissertation, "Reading, Writing, and the Prime Directive: Exploring Emoji as a Literacy Instruction Tool in Developmental Reading and Writing/First Year Writing Corequisites." Petcoff's research study then became part of the work of this volume, written in collaboration with colleagues Janice C. Palaganas and Marcel Danesi.

Their book makes what may be a startling argument to many: that emoji can play a positive instrumental role in teaching and learning. Setting the discussion of emojis within scholarship on semiotics and tracing an historical timeline that connects this contemporary set of symbols to much earlier symbol systems, from hieroglyphics or cave drawings to early comic books, the authors demonstrate that visual modes of communication have been instrumental throughout history as they build a compelling case for taking emojis seriously.

The opening chapter presents a fascinating overview of visual communication and its role in the history of literacy, describes hybrid literacy (emoji plus print) as a "contemporary technologically created mode of integrating verbality and visuality in everyday written communication," explains why an emoji-only form of literacy is unlikely ever to replace traditional systems, and introduces readers to "semioliteracy," a form of literacy "based on the ability to integrate signs selected from any modality to create a message – verbal, visual, audio, and so on." In short, semioliteracy is a hybrid form of writing and reading, a blending of linear phonetic writing with emoji writing in ways that can be very useful in teaching and learning, particularly for scaffolding traditional literacies.

The second chapter offers a review of some of the literature surrounding emoji, sets the discussion of emoji alongside other new forms of literacy (twitteracy, for example), and compares emoji literacy to Ong's discussion of secondary orality and to contemporary arguments for the efficacy of vernacular literacies.

These richly contextual chapters set the scene for the two major case studies treated in this volume, one in a healthcare community and one in a general education program – aimed at demonstrating the pedagogical potential of emojis in the classroom as well as in certain areas of the workforce. These studies are both ingenious in design and rigorous in execution. The Petcoff study revealed that student participants gained a more thorough understanding and awareness of literacy (and literacies), the ability to think critically about their own writing, and the ability to master certain reading and writing requirements. In addition, the use of emoji inspired and supported creativity and helped students understand difficult concepts.

The Palaganas study found that emoji are appearing more and more often in healthcare communications, particularly in healthcare education classroom settings. They are creating controversy and some resistance. This study, then, aims to determine what types of emoji are being used and what attitudes healthcare educators, students, and practitioners hold about them. Not surprisingly, results were mixed and differed according to age, comfort with technology, and so on. Nevertheless, participants associated emoji with expressing emotions, feelings, and greater engagement, suggesting that emoji can "tap into an unconscious need for social bonding, even in professional situations." Thus, they may be increasingly helpful, even for those who may be skeptical of their use.

Throughout, this text is enhanced with the very emoji it studies, helping readers see the symbols at work across a range of rhetorical situations. And while the authors advocate further experiments and research on emoji and are positive in their assessment of the overall contributions emoji literacy can make in and out of the classroom, they are very even-handed in their analysis, considering a range of perspectives and surveying a very large body of literature on the topic. So, whether you are familiar with emoji or not, whether you use them or not, and whatever you think of them, turn the page and begin reading: follow the story of emoji at work and play and see them in the rich historical context offered here. It's my guess you will come away with a lot of new knowledge – and perhaps with more questions than answers.

Indeed, the authors don't claim to have a crystal ball where emoji are concerned, and they certainly don't claim to have all the answers. With impressive humility (and wisdom), they conclude that emoji, after all, are not revolutionary and that they will likely morph into something else or disappear entirely as the technology changes. … It could also well be that emoji bear an unconscious desire that reflects the times – the need to render communication as friendly as possible. In conducting interviews with students, all three authors of this book reported that the overall view that emoji convey a "sunny" tone to human interaction surfaced commonly. It is no accident that the most common emoji bear the color of the sun.

If emoji can shed sunshine, help create understanding among readers and writers, and take some of the tension out of traditional tasks of writing – well, those are good reasons to use them. And good reasons to read this book!

Andrea A. Lunsford
Louise Hewlett Nixon Professor Emerita
Stanford University

Preface

Myriad studies on emoji have come forth since 2015, when the Oxford Dictionary chose as its "Word of the Year" the "Face with Tears of Joy" emoji 😂, catching virtually everyone in the cognitive and communication sciences somewhat off guard. Since then, the role (or more precisely roles) of emoji in routine informal communications has been studied from many disciplinary angles, showing overall that they can no longer be considered to be mere illustrative signs, simply bolstering a message visually. They have become part and parcel of how people communicate in writing on a daily basis, guiding how they conceptualize and structure their messages. Lacking from the ever-broadening research base on the emoji phenomenon are in-depth considerations of how these visual signs can be incorporated practically in areas such as education and healthcare communications. Various studies are starting to show that emoji literacy can aid the realization of learning tasks in education at all levels and help facilitate communications between professionals and the general public, such as interactions between physicians and their patients. As humans, we seem to naturally understand pictures better, which may in itself promote learning. The gist of the studies suggests, in fact, that emoji can complement and even bolster traditional reading and writing skills, making them versatile instructional tools for helping students acquire these skills, especially since emoji, by their very nature, are better understood across cultures, socioeconomic groups, and easily adaptable to different learning levels.

Canadian communications theorist Marshall McLuhan (1962, 1964) had predicted, before the Internet, that an electronic global village, as he named it, had emerged in a world connected by mass communications technologies. In this village, communication would move away gradually from linear print and the written word to nonlinear, visually based, holistic ways of representing information and communicating it across the globe. Nowhere has McLuhan's assessment been more verifiable than it has in the rise of emoji writing. He also predicted that this type of writing would instill into groupthink a form of nonverbal consciousness that would affect how people interacted in everyday life. Everything from education to the perceived value of literacy would change radically. As a consequence, he argued, the new forms of writing and literacy that emerged in the connected globe could not be ignored in areas such as education, since to do so would mean denying children access to the real world and skills that they will need in their future careers.

Our overall objective in writing this book is to follow up on McLuhan's identification of the need to connect the outside world to the classroom, arguing that emoji literacy can no longer be excluded from it. We aim to expand upon the relevant (but sporadic) work of researchers who are finding that emoji are powerful communication tools for the education of children and for facilitating interactions between professionals and their patients or clients. Emoji help students understand and better describe a range of emotions, attitudes, and judgments, which can become the basis for facilitating the acquisition of more intellectual skills, such as traditional academic literacy, perhaps because they attenuate and even obliterate age-old hierarchically based judgments with regard to the backgrounds that students bring to the classroom. They are, simply put, part of a global lingua franca that can bridge the outside world to the inner world of the classroom.

The arguments to be made in this book are based in large part on two empirical research studies conducted by two of the authors of this book (Petcoff and Palaganas), as well as anecdotal studies by the third author (Danesi). All are based on assessing the efficacy of emoji in specific settings and situations. One is centered on a training course for healthcare professionals at the Massachusetts General Hospital Institute of Health Professions, led by Palaganas, a clinician and a professor and lecturer at MGH IHP and Harvard; the other is based on an experiment in literacy training of developmental students, conducted by Petcoff, a literacy instructor. Both have provided insightful results, which are used throughout this book to solidify our overall argument that emoji are key elements in how people communicate and think today. They can no longer be viewed as an ancillary set of picture words for sprucing up informal written messages or a means of projecting the paralinguistic (nonverbal) aspects of oral communication onto the screen. As we will attempt to argue throughout, emoji are learning-enhancing and communication-facilitating devices, with their own semiotic and discursive modalities, that can be applied to both education and profession-based communications profitably.

The book is divided into seven chapters, starting with matters of general concern regarding emoji in Chapter 1. The Petcoff study is summarized and discussed in Chapter 2 and the Palaganas studies in Chapter 4. In between (Chapter 3), we look at the link between education and healthcare communications in a general way – a link that is established by the nature of emoji literacy itself. In Chapters 5 and 6 we develop our arguments for applying emoji to healthcare communications and higher education in general, constituting our primary aim in writing this book. Chapter 7 then distills from the empirical studies the implications they have for emoji theories overall and for their applicability to the educational and healthcare realms. The subtext throughout this book is that the time has come to take advantage of the ability of emoji in such realms to make communication easier and emotively powerful.

We will also intersperse discussions of caveats. Is emoji-based education truly effective? Has it mitigated the literacies of the past, and thus projected education onto a different path than ever before in history? Does it lower the professional register in professional healthcare settings, perhaps demeaning professionalism itself? These questions are actually addressed in an ipso facto fashion by virtue of empirically and qualitatively investigating emoji use in these areas, which constitute a field laboratory for gauging if emoji are indeed effective communicative tools, as well as assaying what possessing emoji literacy itself entails cognitively and emotionally. The overall aim of an "applied emojistics," as it can be called, would be: (1) to describe how emoji contribute (or not) to activating learning processes in students of all backgrounds; (2) to categorize them according to their learning functions according to subject matter; (3) to discuss how they can be incorporated effectively into everyday pedagogy or andragogy; and (4) to investigate what qualities make them effective tools in healthcare communications, especially those involving physician–patient interactions. The questions that applied emojistics raises and aims to investigate, as related to our objectives, are the following: Can empirical knowledge about emoji use be harnessed to enhance learning outcomes and to increase motivation for learning in general? Can the specific modalities of emoji communication enhance clinically based interactions, without impugning their perceived professional integrity? Strangely, there has been little research on these questions. Our goal is to address them directly in this book. We note that in this book the word emoji is used in both its singular and plural meanings.

Where possible, we have used emoji that are Unicode created and part of the accepted Unicode lexicon. In most instances, we use Microsoft's Segoe UI emoji font pictographs because they represent emoji as they are commonly used in texting and other digital communications. In other parts, however, to illustrate emoji's potentiality as a semioliterate tool in education, we have used conceptualized representations of applicable emoji. We have enlisted the aid of graphic artist Elijah Tan to create both the cover art and graphic representations of such emoji. By design (pun intended), Tan's work does not follow the style of the Unicode lexicon, but, as seen on the cover of this book, it is more illustrative in nature. In no way do we intend to assert that these are "real" emoji, in conventional uses. Finally, in an effort to utilize as many standard emoji as possible, there are instances in which we have expressed related healthcare principles and communications by combining standard emoji to do so.

Omonpee W. Petcoff
Janice C. Palaganas
Marcel Danesi
2023

1 The Emoji Phenomenon Reviewed

Prologue

As mentioned in the Preface, it is now a well-known, but still remarkable, fact that in 2015 the Oxford Dictionary's Word of the Year was an emoji – the "face with tears emoji" (Figure 1.1). The dictionary's rationale for this selection was that the emoji was one of the most used new "words" at the time and thus meritorious of its word-of-the-year status.

But what kind of "word" is an emoji? It certainly is not the same kind that an alphabetic word is, which is a representation of the sounds of a spoken word – that is, it stands for its phonemic structure. On the other hand, the term *emoji*, Japanese for "picture word," is a visual sign standing for a referent or concept directly, with no intervening phonemic (or other kind of word-based) representation. Emoji are used typically (if not exclusively) in informal digital texts together with written words – a hybrid mode of writing where both types of words (alphabetic and emoji) are used in a systematically complementary way, semantically and discursively (Danesi 2016; Seargeant 2019).

Since the Oxford Dictionary event, Unicode (an international encoding standard for different scripts) has made a large repertoire of emoji signs available for installation on mobile device keyboards, on apps, and so on, thus allowing for a routinization of hybrid writing and, in some contexts, even the exclusive use of emoji, such as the translation of entire novels into emoji characters. Emoji are visual signs, as mentioned, but they should not be equated with pictographic writing forms, developed over long periods of time, and used

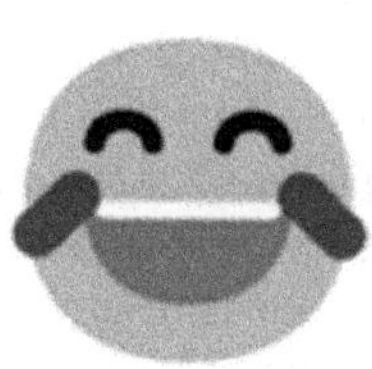

Figure 1.1 Face with tears emoji

in various countries. Emoji are artificially created (or digitally produced) forms that are intended to be language-independent – that is, a user of any language background can select the emoji from preestablished lists to insert within a digital text. As a result, writing now involves two previously separate competencies or literacies – verbal (language-dependent) and visual (generally less dependent on a specific culture, as in art). This has had a broad range of implications for our conceptions of what communication and literacy are, as will be discussed subsequently (Alshenqeeti 2016; Davis 2021; Logi and Zappavigna 2021). Hybrid literacy also has had implications in various domains of society that have traditionally been based on print literacies, including education, which has typically been seen as the channel for imparting and preserving print forms of literacy. Clearly, the advent of emoji into everyday digital discourses has raised some rather profound questions, some of which will be broached initially in this chapter, and examined in more detail in subsequent chapters. The main aim here is to assess the emoji phenomenon generally, including how it has evolved, and what kinds of research findings it has generated. The studies have shown, overall, that emoji signs not only add semantic nuances to messages but also provide a mode of conveying ideas that retrieves visuality as a form of mind. The research has also shown that emoji are not interpreted and used in the same way, as was anticipated by Unicode; rather, like any human semiotic system they involve polysemy, ambiguity, and other variable meaning modalities.

It has become obvious that – at least for the present – emoji can no longer be considered an ancillary set of picture words for sprucing up informal written messages visually. They constitute a veritable discourse and semiotic code, introduced into everyday (informal) communications by digital technologies. As such, they have led to a need to revisit notions such as literacy and communicative competence, as well as what creativity entails, given that using the hybrid code involves an imaginative sense of how to marry verbality and visuality in a blended way, so as to create a unitary account of some message.

Background

As intended by their creators, emoji have spread globally. But they did not arise in a historical vacuum. They would hardly have become part of writing practices in alphabet-using cultures in the first place without various visual-representational trends that took shape in the late nineteenth and early twentieth centuries. One of these was the advent and spread of the comic book, starting in the late 1930s, which blends images and words into a narrative framework. Artistic movements such as Dada and Futurism, among others, also emerged in the first half of the twentieth century, showing that the printed (phonetic) word, laid out in a linear fashion, was losing its supremacy and uniqueness as a mode of representing and communicating thoughts. These conditioned people to become gradually habituated to visual forms as part of representational activities, loosening the grip that print literacy had on society since at least the 1500s.

Emoji writing has retrieved the tendency to represent the world visually, an anthropological fact that is evidenced by the visual images and figures carved or painted on the roofs and walls of ancient caves as well as on artifacts such as vases. These were our earliest picture writings. From the capacity to represent the world visually, ancient writing systems emerged in the first civilizations of the world. These developed three main types of picture signs – pictograms, ideograms, and logograms – before the advent of alphabets. The pictogram stands directly for its referent through some form of resemblance, simulation, or imitation. The degree of resemblance is higher for concrete referents than it is for abstract referents. Abstract referents came to be represented more specifically by ideograms. These also bear resemblance to their referents, but assume much more of a conventional knowledge of the relation between picture and concept on the part of the user. International symbols for such things as public telephones and washrooms today are modern-day descendants of ideographic representation. Over time, as increasingly abstract signs were required, new forms, such as logograms, were developed. These combined elements of pictography and ideography. For example, the Chinese logogram for *east* is a combination of the pictograms for *sun* and *tree*.

Now, in their own artificial way, emoji retrieve the same range of referential modalities of ancient writing systems, albeit highlighting modernized, comic-book (and often humorous) ways of representing concepts, which is what makes them functionally different from the evolutionary forms of picture writing (Table 1.1).

Table 1.1 *Emoji forms and their uses*

Pictograms	These stand directly for their referents by some form of resemblance: simulates in outline form the happy smiling face; represents a (modern-day) house via a schematic resemblance to its structure.
Ideograms	These stand for abstract referents via various degrees of symbolism: alludes to snoring (showing the presumed sounds made in snoring); indicates "being in a hurry," recalling comic-book balloons that represent some sound or action.
Logograms	These combine pictographic and ideographic elements to produce phraseological forms: (I) is a homophonic emoji (*eye* = *I* phonetically); represents a heart (pictographically), which is also used commonly as a symbol for love (ideographically). These require conventional knowledge of the relation between the emoji and its referent. And it is mainly in this domain of reference that emoji produce most of their misinterpretations (to be discussed subsequently).

The scripts of early civilizations eventually developed phonographic elements within them – forms standing for parts of words, such as syllables or individual sounds. A complete phonographic system for representing sounds is the alphabetic one. The first such system emerged in the Middle East and was transported by the Phoenicians to Greece around 1000 BCE. It contained signs for consonant sounds only. In Greece, signs for vowels were added to it, making the Greek system the first full-fledged alphabetic one. The transition from visual to alphabetic writing was not revolutionary; it was evolutionary, developing spontaneously in the marketplaces of the ancient world because it made the writing of transactions rapid and efficient. Every alphabet character is the residue of a stylistic alteration to some earlier visual sign (such as a pictogram). Consider the alphabet character "A" as a case in point. It started out as a pictogram of the head of an ox in Egypt (and other parts of the Middle East). The ox pictogram came, at some point, to be drawn only in its bare outline. It was this outline that came eventually to stand for the word for ox (*aleph*). Around 1000 BCE Phoenician scribes, who wrote from right to left, drew the ox outline sideways (probably because it was quicker for them to do so). The slanted Phoenician figure stood just for the first sound in the word (*aleph*), because it became very familiar. The Greeks, who wrote from left to right, turned the Phoenician figure around the other way. Around 500 BCE, as such "abbreviated picture writing" became more standardized and letters stopped changing directions, the "A" assumed the upright position it has today, derived from Roman script.

Archeologist Schmandt-Besserat (1978, 1992) found that the first commonly used pictographic forms were probably made by clay tokens, which were image-reproducing molds. It is not a stretch to say that the emoji keys on keyboards, websites, and apps are contemporary counterparts of the clay tokens. Actually, the emoji sign system is an endpoint in the evolution of emoticons and kaomoji – respectively, representations of a facial expression such as :-) (smile), formed by various combinations of keyboard characters, and emoticons that use a combination of Japanese characters, Roman alphabet letters, and punctuation marks to represent a facial expression vertically (Evans 2017): (n_n), (^_^), and *(^o^)*, for example.

The psychological difference between alphabetic and emoji script is, as mentioned, a difference between the psychology and semiotics of verbality and visuality, between processing words as discretely composed signs (phonemically) and holistically created signs. The importance of visuality to human knowledge-making and communication was discussed at length by Rudolf Arnheim (1969), who challenged the traditional differentiation between "thinking" (associated with language) and "perceiving" (associated with visual art), claiming that the two have been artificially separated, since they have always co-occurred in human affairs. For Arnheim, visual forms such as paintings are what allow us to have a true understanding of our experiences of the world. In this psychological explanatory framework, it can be argued that emoji have spread so broadly because they have retrieved visuality in everyday communication, used in tandem with other representational structures.

Visuality is assumed to be a more understandable mode than verbality in crosslinguistic and cross-cultural communications, with supposed minimal degrees of interpretive variance. As research by Unicode has shown, facial emoji, designed to resemble facial expressions in suggestive outline form, are the most commonly used ones across the world because of their understandable iconic modalities (that is, their resemblance to facial expressions). But their meanings are not static. For instance, the happy face smiley can be used beyond its initial meaning of happiness to communicate differential connotations and semantic nuances in the context of the intent of a particular message, such as conveying irony. In some countries, such as China, the same emoji might convey mockery instead, given that the eyes on the emoji do not move, as they do on a real face; and this might be interpreted as suppressing a smile, not manifesting it. In the same culture, it could also mean that an interlocutor no longer wants to continue an interaction (Jaeger and Ares 2017). So, while the smiley emoji is assumed to be conducive to a straightforward interpretation, no matter what native language interlocutors speak, it reveals an inherent law of semiotics – diversity in interpretation is a product of using all sign forms. Nevertheless, this emoji (and most other facial emoji) has had a broad acceptance across the world, indicating that its intended meaning becomes accepted broadly, by force of constant intercultural usage, reflecting a kind of semiotic law of normalization via pragmatic utilization.

Specific design strategies to make the emoji code as universally understandable and culturally neutral as possible were adopted initially. For example, the use of yellow to color most of the facial emoji and the deployment of nondistinct facial signifiers (standing for the mouth, the eyes, facial shape, and the eyebrows) were stylistic attempts intended, arguably, to remove recognizable facial features associated with human diversity. But, almost right after the spread of the emoji code into common usage, Unicode was criticized for not reflecting the diversity of its users. So, new facial emoji, including color options, were designed on purpose to reflect culturally based, ethnically sensitive, and gender-flexible referents. Interpretive variance is manifest especially among the ideographic and logographic emoji; but it can also occur in pictographic forms. For example, the emoji of an airplane could be interpreted as referring to the plane itself, flying, traveling, or being at an airport. One cannot assume an isomorphic relation between the emoji and its anticipated interpretation, even by speakers of the same language, and even within the constraints imposed on interpretation by context. Differential interpretations of the same emoji might also be shaped by the platform used – two people looking at a facial emoji on different platforms might interpret it differently.

A now famous example of misinterpretation due to platform-based variance occurred in 2020, when British actress Jameela Jamil posted a tweet using the face-with-hand-over-mouth emoji as a social commentary on food-challenged people shopping during the coronavirus pandemic (Rathore 2022). On Apple's iOS, the emoji conveys a pensive (worried) feeling state, but on other platforms it appeared as a giggling face, leaving many receivers of the tweet upset, believing that Jamil was mocking poor people, even though this was not her intended meaning.

The ways in which the emoji code generates meaning have been examined across disciplines since 2015. The gist of the work indicates that they provide a grid of visual-holistic meanings that guides the interpretation of a hybrid message, constituting an annotative template to its meaning. Some work suggests that they project the "body language" that accompanies face-to-face interaction onto the screen. While this is not the only function of emoji, it does seem to have plausibility in some uses. In this area, David McNeill's notion of *gesticulants* (1992, 2005), which he adopted from Adam Kendon (1972), is a useful one. These are spontaneous co-speech gestures that depict the content of utterances, bringing out images that cannot be shown overtly in verbal speech, as well as the mental images of what the speaker is thinking about.

McNeill subdivided gesticulants into five main categories, against which various emoji can be mapped:

(1) *Iconic*: These mirror or simulate in gestural form what is being said. Common examples are the circular hand movements when talking about roundabout reasoning, moving the hands far apart when talking of something large, moving both the head and hands in an upward direction when saying "Let's go up," and so on. Emoji standing for iconic gesticulants are common:

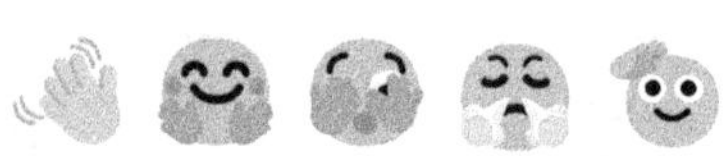

(2) *Metaphoric*: These are accompanying gestures that depict the image schemas underlying metaphorical utterances. Examples are the kinds of gesticulants that are used spontaneously with conduit metaphors, with the hands put forward as if they are passing on something to someone or receiving something from someone – "presenting an idea," "putting forth an argument," "offering advice," "give it to me," "this is for me," and so on. Again, note that the emoji is not always isomorphic to the physical gesticulant but portrays the concept behind it. Below are a few examples:

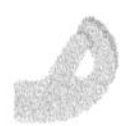

"*That* is the point!"

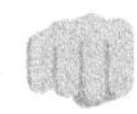

"You got it!"

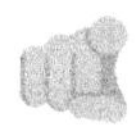

"*You* are the problem"

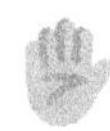

"Hold up a sec"

(3) *Beat*: This is a gesticulant involving hand actions that resemble the beating of musical tempo, whereby speakers flick a hand or fingers up and down, or back and forth, to accompany the rhythmic pulsation of speech. Beats mark the introduction of new concepts in an utterance. They are used commonly when "making points" – "first … second … and lastly"; or in phrases such as "let me repeat this," which is rendered visually by the emoji below; note that some linguists suggest that any repeating emoji has a beat function, which is plausible in certain contexts, but can be ambiguous in this kind of repetitive form. The emoji below are simple examples of beat gesticulants:

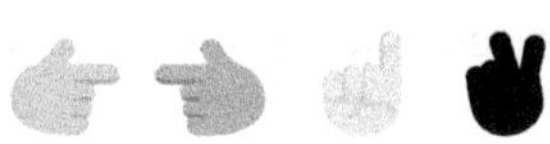

(4) *Cohesive*: Cohesive gesticulants involve using the hands to emphasize that the separate parts of an utterance hold together. They also are used to signal that an utterance is coming to an end or a conclusion, or else that the interlocutor should listen to the final words, as the following emoji imply:

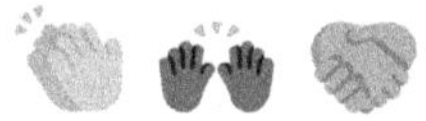

(5) *Deictic*: Hand actions that indicate something that had been mentioned earlier in a conversation, such as waving a hand near the ear and shoulder to indicate that something has passed, are called deictic. These can also be indexes meant to point out (emphasize) something conceptually, as the following common emoji (which also have sign functions, used on walls or devices) indicate:

McNeill's gesticulant categories are subtypes of illustrators (Efron 1941; Ekman 2003). They can be defined generically as instinctive co-speech gestural movements that illustrate the content (literal and metaphorical) of vocal utterances. As such, they provide a basis for studying how gesture and language form a single integrated system in verbal discourse. However, gesticulant emoji are actually not like the physical ones that instinctively accompany speech, as emoji are selected intentionally to convey a concept, not instinctively as in hand gesturing. As such, their gesticulant functions are sporadic, rather than systematic.

Because emoji are used across languages and by individuals of all backgrounds, with varying degrees of traditional literacy, they present themselves as highly useful and inclusive teaching devices, since they involve no assumptions as to literacy background. This aspect has led to a research study on the part of one of the authors of this book (Petcoff 2023) whereby emoji were used as tokens to impart literacy to learners with developmental challenges. The findings and implications will be discussed in the next chapter. Suffice it to say here that using emoji with other digital signs constitutes an out-of-classroom literacy that can easily be brought into the classroom as a pedagogical metalanguage through which literacy training can unfold. It is an example of using the known to reach the unknown via a form of inductive transference, whereby developmental reading and writing students can unconsciously reflect upon how language can be used for academic expressive reasons with the emoji code (Gee 1989; Street 2003; Lea and Street 2006). The Petcoff study showed that emoji literacy can be incorporated pedagogically and andragogically to help students achieve academic literacy, because emoji writing taps directly into the communicative habits of the students, thus operationalizing it as a practical language of instruction in view of laying a path toward a broader form of literacy, as required by schools and society.

Discourse and Semiotic Functions

It is useful to divide the main, or meta, functions of emoji into discourse and semiotic ones – the former refers, simply, to the communicative aspects of emoji use and the latter to the meaning structures and interpretive range of emoji; but in most uses the two overlap considerably. A primary function is the phatic one (Malinowski 1923; Jakobson 1960) – speech used for ritualistic interaction and for keeping social bonds intact or lubricated. For example, a happy face smiley used at the beginning of a text message has the same intent of verbal salutations such as "Hello," "Dear so-and-so," and the like. But it does much more than this – it provides an opening interpretive frame for imbuing the tone of the message with positivity, thus ensuring that a phatic bond between interlocutors is established. On the other hand, in a conflictual message, the same emoji would indicate an ironic or sarcastic intent, providing a different interpretive frame for grasping the function of the entire message. This shows how the discourse and semiotic functions can overlap, depending on intent, which is what makes emoji semiotically and discursively powerful.

Another primary function is the emotive one. This is the portrayal (consciously or unconsciously) of the emoji user's state of mind, mood, attitude, and so on; the desired effect on the receiver that the emoji is designed to have is called the conative function. In face-to-face communication, people use interjections, intonation, and other prosodic strategies, alongside specific words and phrases, to convey their feelings, explicitly or implicitly, and as strategies to elicit reactions in interlocutors. In hybrid digital messages, these functions are rendered by sentiment-based emoji such as faces, hearts, and the like. However, it can be said that the emotive-conative functions are built into virtually every emoji, given that they are chosen not to convey literal information, but to inject emotional tone and semantic nuances into a message. So, a heart emoji placed at the start of a message will tend to imbue the message with "heart-felt" nuances, whether these are authentic or feigned for satirical reasons (Danesi 2022). The emoji code can thus be said to constitute a "sentiment-placement-based distributive system" – that is, a means to infuse an entire message with sentiment by placing appropriate emotively charged emoji at strategic locations in a message so as to shape the message in terms of intent and emotivity, on both parts. This can be called an "episodic" structure, which is different from verbal syntax or style in the fact that the placement of the emoji signs is not governed by rules of syntax, but rather by unconscious rules of emotivity; that is, emoji are placed in strategic locations among the episodes of a text to inform its meaning in terms of these emoji insertions.

What characterizes an emotive-episodic representational system is that the emotions or moods injected into a message are left unnamed and must be gleaned through the visuality system of understanding (Novak et al. 2015). A key study by Cohn and colleagues (2018) found that emoji placement was not subject to the normal rules of grammar. The researchers examined the type and location of emoji (within clauses, at the start, and at the end), finding that there was a "processing cost" for deciphering images as compared to words – that is, it took more time for subjects to process the meaning of emoji when compared to word placement, determined by syntax, indicating a different mode of processing emoji versus words. However, the kind of implicit knowledge that emoji placement implies indicated that there was no significant difference in comprehensibility between word and congruent-image placements.

Another function of emoji is illustrative, reinforcing the contents of a message via imagery (emoji of a house, a car, etc.); however, even in such uses the emotive-episodic modality built into emoji involves the injection of annotative nuances to their placement. The meaning of "really looking forward to

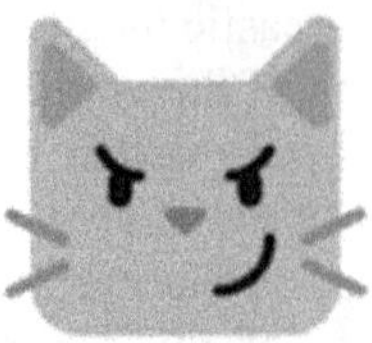

Figure 1.2 Ironic cat face emoji

the meeting" changes significantly when accompanied by an eye-rolling emoji, which adds an ironic annotation to the message (Robson 2019). The cat-face-with-a-wry-smile emoji is an example of how an emoji can be placed episodically in a text to imply irony or mockery visually, no matter what the content may be, evoking the same pattern of understanding that characterizes the decoding of verbal irony (Weissman and Tanner 2018; Figure 1.2).

The choice of a cat (with a wry facial grin) as suggesting irony is consistent with one of the perceived roles of cats in cartoons, comics, and literary traditions. The cat emoji can be traced, arguably, to the figure of the Cheshire Cat – the fictional cat made popular by Lewis Carroll in his children's novel, *Alice's Adventures in Wonderland* (1865). Carroll's cat has become known for its distinctive mischievous grin, which is left as a trace after the Cat's periodic and gradual disappearances. This suggests that an emoji does not sever its connectivity to previous connotative meanings.

Another major function involves the use of emoji as projections of the prosodic-tonal features of face-to-face discourse onto the written text (Evans 2017). In effect, these emoji are body language signs; but they too have episodic function since they can also guide the desired interpretation of a message when placed at certain locations – encoding a mood or sentiment that is distributed into other parts of the message. So, if the intended sentiment is "unhappiness," then, say, a facial emoji with a frown and closed, downcast eyes, simulating sorrow or pain (😔), might be used in places where this sentiment is evoked. This sentiment then becomes part of the subtext of the entire message, leaving its emotive traces episodically (Danesi 2022). Analogously, facial emoji that project humor, pensiveness, contradiction, uncertainty, and the like onto the written message have episodic-distributive functions.

One discourse function that is seemingly missing from emoji use, given that they are employed primarily in informal communications, are the normal sociolinguistic registers – modes of communicating that are designed to match the formality of a situation, the medium used, or the nature of the topic involved in a speech act. In an emoji-using text many of the sociolinguistic categories (register, honorifics, etc.) collapse, or at the very least are not marked as they are in routine communications. This does not mean that they cannot be used to convey politeness. This will be discussed subsequently within the healthcare communications field, where politeness is an expected feature of the interactions.

As mentioned earlier, one of the primary functions of emoji (especially the facial ones) is to reproduce facial microexpressions, according to speech act typologies (Searle 1969, 1976), rendering them, however, in humorous-cartoonish ways. A microexpression is a facial expression that lasts briefly, resulting from an emotional response to something. A leading researcher on microexpressions is American psychologist Paul Ekman, a notion he adapted from the key work of Haggard and Isaacs (1966) and Hjortsjö (1970), adding significant detail to it. Perhaps the reason why facial emoji tend to be the ones most used across the world, and the ones generating less meaning variance, is because they are designed according to universal microexpressions. Ekman and his co-researchers (Ekman and Friesen 1971; Ekman 1989; Matsumoto 1992) found a high level of consistency in various cultures in how they identified the basic microexpressions in virtually identical ways for basic emotions such as embarrassment, anxiety, guilt, pride, relief, contentment, pleasure, shame, and a few others. Illustrative examples of microexpression emoji are shown below:

- "I am pretty sure that this is fishy": 
- "Trust me, this is correct":  
- "This is disgusting": 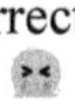 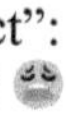
- "This is hilarious": 
- "This is amazing!": 
- "I am not amused": 
- "What a relief!": 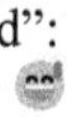
- "This is becoming boring": 
- "What an embarrassment": 

The list of such microexpression emoji is endless, and it is being constantly updated and expanded for various speech act functions. The semiotic problem with these (and most other emoji) is that culturally shaped meaning variance crops up from time to time that may lead to misinterpretations in messages. The thumbs-up emoji, , which is still identified as one of the most used emoji across the world, is now a widely known case in point, since the gesture it represents has a whole array of unwanted connotations that users in some non-English speaking countries want to avoid, finding the emoji derogatory or insulting.

Some microexpression emoji are used as gambits – words or phrases used to open a conversation, to keep it going, to make it smooth, to repair any anomaly within it, and so on. The following are common English gambits with corresponding emoji:

- "Uh huh … yeah … hmm … aha … ": 
  This gambit is a filler, allowing an interlocutor to make it known to the other interlocutor that they are in fact in agreement as the message proceeds. The smiley emoji repeated in sequence suggests encouragement to keep an idea being expressed going.
- "I didn't say that": 
  Negation can be represented in various ways with different kinds of emoji, depending on the intensity desired.
- "You like this, don't you?": 
  Tag questions ensure consent. The thumbs-up emoji is one way to insert the tag question gambit in a message, albeit with reservations as to the meaning of the thumbs-up gesture (as mentioned).
- "May I ask you something?": 
  Questions designed to gain entry into a conversation can be rendered by various emoji. This one indicates that a thought has come into the interlocutor's mind (during a repartee) suggesting the desire to interject something into the digital conversation.
- "No way!": 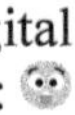
  Forceful interjections indicate agreement or disagreement patterns during a conversation. The emoji shows how this gambit can be realized in a lighthearted, wry way.

It is to be emphasized that the gambit-focused microexpression emoji selected above reflect subjective choices; indeed, many other emoji could have been chosen to communicate the same type of utterance. This suggests that emoji, like verbal language, vary idiolectally or subjectively (for example, Dainas and Herring 2021).

A salient feature of emoji in general is that they compress meaning efficiently, thus increasing the economy of conversational sequences. One or two emoji can, for instance, be used to answer a question such as: "How are you?" (a happy face emoji, a sad face emoji, a thumbs-up or thumbs-down emoji, etc.). Such one-or-two-emoji responses not only economize on the verbal structural material that would otherwise be required but also minimize the exchange of perfunctory repartees, making communication more efficient and less prone to interactive superfluity. Moreover, the one-or-two-emoji response can fill in gaps of meaning that might otherwise emerge in the course of a communication, often signaled verbally by expressions such as "I am not quite sure how to say this" or "I can't find the right word." This implies, more generally, that emoji might be able to combat manifestations of hypocognition, or the inability to communicate certain ideas because there are either no words for them or else the appropriate words cannot be found (Levy 1975).

Interestingly, it has been found that when we look at a smiley face, the same parts of the brain are activated as when we look at a real human face (for example, Churches et al. 2014). While emoji are communicatively efficient when used alone, a study by Scheffler and colleagues (2021) has shed considerable light on how the emotive content of emoji is processed. Subjects were asked to read texts with emoji in them, as the researchers measured the reading time they used to do so precisely. As expected, it took them a little longer to comprehend a sentence that includes emoji than one that does not. This extra time implies that the brain is mapping the emoji against the content of the message via processes that are not unlike those employed in figurative language processing, whereby a concrete referent (for example, *sweet*) is mapped onto an abstract one (for example, *love*) to produce a metaphorical thought: *love is sweet*. The presence of metaphorical meaning in emoji interpretation is a constant one. As Regina Robson remarks (2019): "There is no literal meaning. Emoji are frequently used as a substitution for text, such as inserting multiple hearts in lieu of writing 'love.'" While comprehending a hybrid message of text and emoji may be a bit more time-consuming, the meaning of the message is more easily and clearly understood during processing, as if speaking to someone in person.

Part of the process of unpacking the meaning of emoji involves deciphering pairing sequences, that is, the interpretation of emoji used in combination with other emoji or specific words and phrases – a feature called adjacency pairing in discourse study (Halliday 1985). Common adjacency pairings in digital messages include the following:

- The smiley happy face, the heart emoji, and the thumbs-up emoji often appear alongside phrases such as "That's true," "I agree"; but they also surface contrastively with statements such as "That's really not true" and "I wouldn't say that."
- The hand-clapping emoji, the hands raised in celebration emoji, and the handshaking emoji are found commonly alongside phrases such as "Yeah," "Sure," "Right"; but also contrastively (ironically) with "No-no," "No way," "Not true," and the like.
- The thinking face emoji (with the hand touching the chin), the side eye emoji, and the emoji face with a finger pointing to the head are found frequently alongside disagreement statements such as "Yeah, but, maybe."
- Tag questions, such as "You agree, don't you?," are commonly accompanied by emoji clusters such as the question mark followed by consent emoji.

As Wagner et al. (2020) have noted, the hidden power of emoji communication is that it can "fundamentally alter the exchange of emotion [because] images and signs that depict feelings have replaced the nuanced selection of the right words and phrases." As the authors go on to surmise: "Across the globe, the expressive range of human emotion through the static ideogram of the emoji, or emoticon, presents an increasing challenge for the visually immediate, nonverbal exchange of capricious emotive communication."

Hybrid Literacy

One of the central questions raised by emoji writing regards the conceptualization of the notion of literacy, which, in its broadest sense, is the expression of thoughts in written form in some conventionalized way. Since the first civilizations, literacy competence has formed the basis for both official and informal communications in written form. As such, it is something that is passed on in educational settings, so as to provide young learners with the writing and reading skills that might be required by a society in most of its formal activities, from law to science and historiography. The actual features considered to be part of literacy will, however, vary from one society to another, within which there may also be the need to impart other kinds of literacies – numerical literacy, for example. But, generally speaking, literacy implies the capacity required to create and comprehend written texts that are perceived as critical for competent membership in a society.

Stories have always been seen as crucial for imparting literacy during childhood. The term *emergent literacy* (Clay 1966) is sometimes used to refer to the child's knowledge of what reading a story implies, whereby the child can reiterate story lines and character descriptions meaningfully, connecting them to the printed words of the story, thus connecting writing to the development of concepts. In many children's stories, verbal literacy is linked to visual representation, via illustrations in storybooks that function as not only illustrators but also visual annotations and episodic signs that allow the child to integrate written text with conceptualizations. Known as picture books, these involve hybrid composition, where the visual images help children gain literacy. One could say that these books are precursors to the hybrid writing styles of today, where instead of artist-created images, emoji are selected by the writers themselves to similarly make their messages effective via the blending of text and images. Research on picture books (for example Hsiao 2010) has shown that they improve children's overall literacy, stimulating their engagement with books and literacy more generally. The same technique can be seen today throughout the digital world, with written texts composed as amalgams of print with visual and animated structures, which make websites and digital presentations much more understandable.

Hybrid literacy (emoji plus print) is clearly not something new; as such, it is a contemporary technologically created mode of integrating verbality and visuality in everyday written communications. Because of its ubiquity, we no longer perceive such writing as exceptional or, on the other side, as destructive of traditional literacy. Rather, we now see it as a way to communicate effectively and creatively to express and react to messages. Hybrid literacy has thus eliminated, or at the very least attenuated, the traditional distinction between separate verbal and nonverbal literacies. As Halliday (1985: 82) predicted a while back: "When new demands are made on language, it changes in response to them. We are making language work for us in ways it never had to do before, it will have to become a different language in order to cope." All this raises, however, an obvious question: Has the kind of print literacy that has served us so well in the past lost its value and functions? Marshall McLuhan (1962) predicted that the global village connecting people electronically, as he named it, would look both forward and backward – forward to a form of literacy that involved nonlinear modes of representing information and backward to an age when visual writing emerged as the first form of literacy, in Sumer, Egypt, China, and other areas of the world. Nowhere is McLuhan's assessment more verifiable than it is in the rise of hybrid writing.

It should be mentioned at this point that some have proposed an emoji-only form of literacy, to completely replace the traditional print-based form. But this is unlikely because it would violate one of the well-known psychological laws of communication – namely, that communicative systems evolve along of the path of least effort (Zipf 1935, 1949), and thus, as a corollary, any written text that is effortful to decipher for various reasons is unlikely to become part and parcel of communicative-representational practices. One of the first books to be translated completely into emoji is *Emoji Dick*, by Fred Berenson, in 2009, a complete emoji version of *Moby Dick*. The problem with reading this version is that without knowing the verbal text, it is truly effortful to even piece the images together into a narrative frame, most of which could be interpreted in a variety of ways that have little to do with the novel. So, what arguably hampers the spread of such writing is the kind of effort required to decipher emoji-only texts.

Given the commonality of hybrid literacy, the question of whether or not such literacy can be used to impart reading and writing skills in classroom settings, given that it taps directly into students' communicative competence, is hardly a moot one, as work by Petcoff (2023) has shown, which discovered how hybrid literacy can be transferred to the acquisition of traditional academic literacy (i.e., chapter 2). The premise is the same one undergirding the use of picture books to impart literacy to children – namely, awareness of how language can be used to express ideas emerges much more easily in subjects who have little or no background in print literacy itself. As Lu et al. (2016: 270) have observed:

> From a human-computer interaction perspective, emoji have significant advantages over plain text in facilitating the communication of smartphone users. The compactness of emoji reduces the effort of input; the rich semantics they convey expresses ideas and emotions more vividly; emoji do not have language barriers, making it possible to communicate among users from different countries. These advantages have attributed to the popularity of emoji all over the world, making them a "ubiquitous language" that bridges everyone.

Students whose background literacy challenges constitute a learning obstacle will likely gain very little from being exposed to traditional literacy-imparting pedagogy in the classroom. Various reasons for this could be put forward, but one that resonates semiotically is Susanne Langer's (1937: 18) differentiation of discursive, nondiscursive, and presentational modes of understanding, whereby she contended that a visual mode of expression, such as art, is highly effective because it is what she called presentational (understood holistically without breaking it up into its components), whereas the print (textual) mode requires such breaking up. She called this the discursive mode. Discursivity can apply to symbols other than words – it is a mode of expression and understanding based on arrangement with stable and contextualized meanings into a new meaning. Presentational expression operates independently of fixed and stable elements – it does not involve building up an understanding of the elements in a text in isolation; it is understood as a whole. For example, an element used in one painting may be used to represent an entirely different meaning in another. It is this internal contextualization of elements that led her to maintain that "form could be abstracted logically" from content (Langer 1950: 520).

Semioliteracy

The preceding discussion implies several key issues, which will be addressed in this book: How can knowledge of the hybrid writing system be incorporated andragogically (as well as pedagogically) as a way to impart literacy, especially in the case of adult learners? We focus on two very different areas to explore how emoji facilitate communication: learners with developmental needs as well as those involved in healthcare communications. The former explores how emoji are used as a teaching tool; the latter explores the general use of emoji as communicative tools in a specific area of discourse.

The overall principle adopted here is that by using emoji in teaching about literacy, students will not only acquire the ability to grasp the discursive structures involved in literate expression but also be able to use their emoji competence (presentational knowledge) freely to make the path toward gaining literacy a more fluid one. As the Petcoff study has shown, students gain a concrete understanding of the functions of signs (verbal or visual) in their most meaningful (everyday usage) contexts, becoming adept at integrating presentational, discursive, and recursive sign structures to read and write – recursion is used here to mean the repeated application of some structural form or process in different contexts as part of various communicative functions. In textual writing, subject and object pronouns, locative particles, demonstratives, adverbs, and other kinds of so-called deictic forms are recursive structures referencing other parts of speech. Recursive emoji are found constantly in messages, indicating that they have blended distributive and episodic functions (discussed subsequently). Suffice it to say here that they are episodic structures; their insertion in different message locations makes reference to some concept stated before (anaphoric reference) or to some anticipated concept (cataphoric reference). So, if a heart emoji is used before the statement, "I love you," then it is anaphoric; if it is used after, it is a kind of mnemonic device that functions cataphorically.

Given that emoji involve a blend of discursive and semiotic functions, as already discussed, their utilization falls more precisely under the theoretical framework of *semioliteracy* (Petcoff 2022a, 2022b, 2023), a form of literacy based on the ability to integrate signs selected from any modality to create a message – verbal, visual, audio, and so on. Such literacy is now an unconscious one, given the presence of all kinds of sign forms and systems, from emoji to animations to picture memes, that can be used to compose messages. So, the term semioliteracy embraces all kinds of literacies *in actu* and is thus key to devising pedagogically appropriate literacy instruction tools. As McLuhan (1962) argued, writing practices are based on a specific technology (writing tools) that is shaped evolutionarily by other technologies (such as the printing press). This does not mean shedding previous notions of literacy; on the contrary, it means integrating them with current technologically based literacies. By coordinating traditional literacy with the new literacies, the semioliteracy approach in teaching will allow teachers to tap into ever-evolving student learning styles, so as to balance these with the curricular standards set forth by learning institutions and governing bodies. Within this organic context, the definition of semioliteracy actually matches the definition of literacy put forth by UNESCO as "the ability to identify, understand, interpret, create, communicate and compute, using printed and written materials associated with varying contexts" (Montoya 2018).

Concretely, semioliteracy is the ability to comprehend and utilize signs of all kinds (presentational, discursive, recursive) in any technological modality (verbal, visual, audio, animated, etc.) in terms of contextual constraints mapped against traditional forms of print literacy. It encompasses the ability to cultivate an overall semiotic-discursive competence that is required in today's complex technological world. Within the semioliteracy theoretical framework, it is the hybrid form of writing and reading – a blending of linear phonetic writing with emoji writing – that forms the central approach to instruction. This approach can also be called *bimodal*, which provides a neuroscientific slant on the pattern of integration that is implied by the combined use of verbality and visuality in writing (Chapter 2). The effectiveness of the semioliterate approach was investigated by Petcoff with a group of developmental reading and writing students at Tarrant County College Southeast Campus in Arlington, Texas. While the Texas Higher Education Coordinating Board defines the general criteria for identifying developmental reading and writing students and schools across Texas, each school was allowed to implement its own relevant instructional programs. One particular model – the Integrated Reading and Writing Model, mandated by the THEC Board – addresses situations where the acquisition and mastery of literacy prove to be more challenging to developmental learners. The semioliteracy framework adopted by Petcoff afforded her an opportunity to circumvent the usual challenges to literacy acquisition that such learners face. But its implications reach beyond, since it can be argued that it is beneficial to students of all backgrounds and needs.

The term semioliteracy actually encapsulates educational-instructional practices that have been developed since the rise of technologically based literacies and thus constitutes a broad rubric for discussing and examining learning outcomes. Already in 2011, Jody Shipka, an English professor at the University of Maryland, introduced a model for operationalizing multimodal literacy as a blend of digital and non-digital modes of expression. As Shipka (2011) claimed, the distinction between technical (formal) or nontechnical (nonformal) literacy is losing its value in a multimodal world of mass communications. However, she cautions that those who over-enthusiastically adopt digitized texts or computerized teaching tools exclusively as a means of practicing multimodal teaching are shortsighted, given that such training fails to take into account the academic literacy that is still required today. As she argues, multimodality does not involve exclusion of print literacy but rather its amalgamation with the other multimodal literacies reemerging in the world, and is used in tandem with other modes of conveying information. One of her most seemingly bizarre, yet pointedly relevant, examples of her overall approach is her use of pink ballet slipper shoes to teach multimodal composition (Shipka 2011: 1), as part of what she calls "three dimensional" teaching, whereby the shoes involve meaning exchanges that are relevant to the students, given that they can relate to them semiotically – that is, they are perceived as part of a system of understanding that integrates language, objects, social functions, and so on into a type of instruction that brings elements of the real world into the abstract system of understanding called the classroom. Shipka uses the slippers in the classroom to allow students to envision them as objects (in the semiotic sense) that become a basis of discussion. As (Shipka 2011: 7) notes, overall:

> If we are committed to creating courses that provide students with opportunities to forge new connections, to work in highly flexible ways, and to be increasingly cognizant of the ways texts provide shape for and take shape from the contexts in which they are produced, circulated, valued, and responded to, it is crucial … that we not limit the range of materials or technologies students might take up later in compelling ways.

Shipka's approach is fundamentally a semioliterate one, and as such it was adopted and adapted by Petcoff, formerly a special education teacher in the Arlington Independent School District and current developmental reading and writing college instructor (Chapter 2). Above all else, she found that this approach reverberated emotionally and intellectually with underprivileged and othered students. The resources to teach them are not as plentiful as those earmarked for the mainstream classroom. So, the developmental reading and writing instructor has always been faced with the need to create self-styled teaching tools from whatever resource is available. Using emoji to teach literacy skills implies providing, at the very least, a repertory of pedagogical techniques and materials for addressing the learning issues that traditional publishers have tended to ignore. As with Shipka's pink ballet shoes, emoji are effective semiotically because they resonate with the students at different levels of understanding. They offer a means to present abstract concepts via familiar visual signs. Also like the Shipka approach, different media and semiotic sign systems are mapped onto the core emoji-literacy approach, including video, mobile phones, popular culture texts, and so on, so as to create a multimodal learning environment that mirrors and reproduces the communicative environment in which the students find themselves immersed on a daily basis.

Although emoji meanings may vary across cultures and according to operating systems or web platforms, overall, the emoji code comprises a recognizable visual code that is used throughout the world. Traditional literacy instruction tools were crafted on the basis of alphabetic texts, with proficiency and mastery involving the ability to perform basic decoding and encoding processes on such texts. While these skills are certainly needed today, the discursive nature of traditional literacy instruction does not allow learners today to gain access to the structures of print literacy, given that they are constrained in function (to academic texts); and moreover, as media such as YouTube now show, multimodality can no longer be avoided, even in literacy education, since people have become accustomed to seeing, hearing, and reading information traditionally available only in text (Selfe 2017).

In sum, the semioliteracy framework aims to integrate different sign systems into a coherent holistic model of what understanding texts implies today. It is the core notion in what is called *edusemiotics* (Semetsky and Stables 2014) – a pedagogical approach in which teaching any subject matter should take into direct account the semiotic notions that undergird sign use. As a simple, yet nontrivial example, teaching math literacy in an edusemiotic way would involve presenting: (1) the signs necessary to carry out some task or to conceptualize some idea, (2) using some visual-semiotic strategy to make ideas more comprehensible, and (3) comparing mathematical signs with other kinds of signs so as to bring out common principles of representation. This is not new, of course, but it was never named as a specific kind of approach. So, the usual diagrams used in mathematics can be seen to be edusemiotic tools in that they present information concretely, and thus much more comprehensibly, by highlighting or showing the essential features of a problem. As Richard Skemp (1971: 101) has put it, a diagram "conveys all that verbal statements do, more clearly and vividly." In a sense, emoji are the equivalent of mathematical diagrams, since they present information clearly and vividly.

Other components of a semioliteracy-based pedagogy involve reader-transactional theory, media/digital literacy, multimodal composition, and visual literacy. Transactional theory, developed by Louise Rosenblatt (for example, Rosenblatt 2005), proposes that teaching a learner to read involves both the reader and the text itself in the conceptualization of its meaning – not their separation into distinctive components. The meaning extracted from a text is, therefore, produced by a continuous transaction between the reader and the text, involving above all else the experiential background a reader brings to the text. This shift of focus onto the reader has been a trend within semiotics proper. The late Umberto Eco (1979) was among the first to indicate that there is a relation between how a text is interpreted in any era and the nature of the interpreters themselves. Successful interpretation of the text on the part of a reader is not a straightforward matter of trying to determine the text-maker's intentions, but invariably involves what is in the reader's mind at the outset. In effect, there is a negotiation of meaning between text-maker and reader that ends up in varying interpretations across social systems and across time. Given their episodic nature, emoji can be used as particular kinds of interpretive frames in text analysis, since they allow for annotation and commentary on the print text via their visual nature, again, much like the illustrations in picture books. This view of texts has shattered the traditional critical approach to interpretation assigned to those with specialized literacy (such as critics), opening textual analysis up to anyone, anywhere (Freire 1970; Bourdieu 1972). The semioliteracy pedagogical model can be summarized as seen in Figure 1.3.

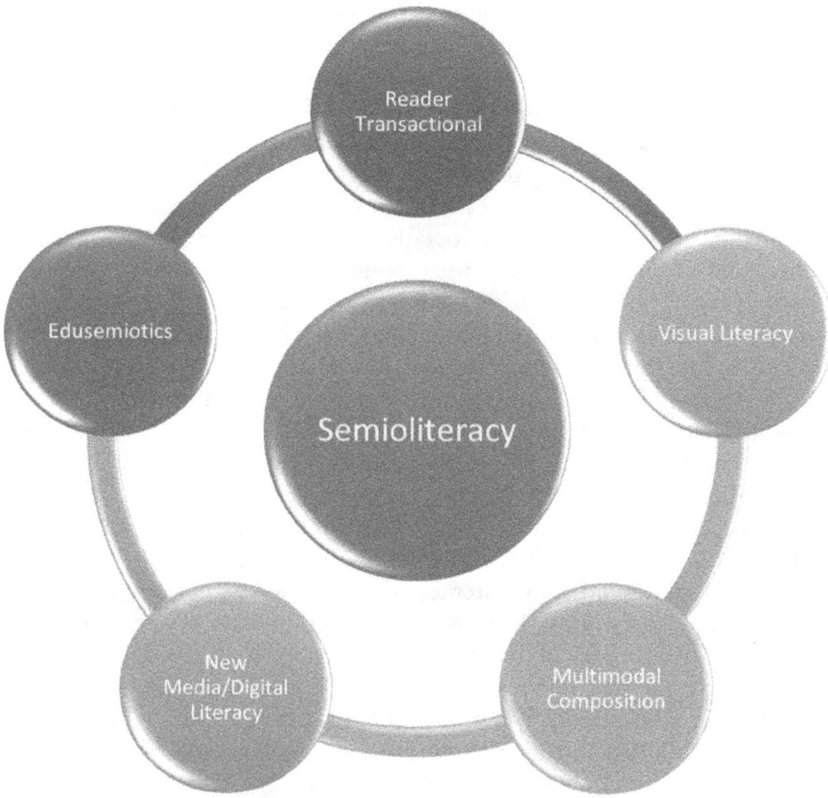

Figure 1.3 Semioliteracy

This model is intended to take into account diversity of learning styles, background variables, and various other aspects that aim to make textual analysis truly open to everyone. One of the first to realize that semioliteracy was critical in activating learning was the semiotician-psychologist Lev Vygotsky (1961), who put forth the idea of "zones of proximal development," implying that learners progress through zones of learning that become extended spontaneously as soon as they are able to understand new input by themselves. He proposed developmental stages that go from external (physical and social) actions toward internal cognitive representations that find expression in the diverse semiotic activities (verbal and nonverbal). As such, he saw a coordination of different literacies as key to the acquisition of knowledge and skill. The student is thus a "creator of knowledge," rather than a passive consumer. As Shafer (1998: 19) characterizes such approaches, pedagogical optimization is realized when students are allowed to learn "through a gradual and constructive approach." In the area of literacy instruction, the central idea is to show that reading and writing are not just academic skills, but social and technologically shaped ones as well. While emoji themselves are not marked for register (discussed subsequently), they nonetheless can be used as an access route to the higher registers implied by possessing print literacy.

The movement known as "new literacies studies" took shape in the 1980s as one of the first to put forth a socially based semioliteracy approach at the threshold of the digital age (for example, Gee 2015). In contrast to traditional literacy pedagogy, which envisioned reading and writing as an abstract (idealistic) process inside the mind, the members of the movement argued that literacy was something we did in society, not just inside our heads, and should be taught and studied as such. It viewed literacy as a sociocultural rather than just a mental phenomenon. A supporter of this view, Brian Street (2013), put forth a derived model that he calls, "autonomous literacy instruction," in which he suggests that literacy outside of any social context is meaningless because it is abstract and self-serving and, thus, is nonfunctional. The main problem with traditional literacy instruction is that the technical functions of literacy are presented as being independent of any concrete social uses. The rote memorization of rules and patterns in reading, writing, and discursive practices is encouraged in a decontextualized fashion, rendering literacy as largely pointless. While Street sees the role of technical knowledge (grammar, phonics, style, etc.) as important, he stresses that it should be taught from a context-dependency point of view, so that the teacher can illustrate the importance of "the broader cultural perception of ways of thinking about and doing reading and writing in cultural contexts at work" (Street 2003).

In line with the traditional sociosemiotic view of language (including Vygotsky and Halliday), linguist James Paul Gee (2015) sees literacy instruction as needing to be connected with contemporaneous social needs and communicative patterns. In other words, literacy makes sense if it is mapped against actual communicative practices. It is in this framework that a semioliteracy approach that incorporates emoji as a nontraditional literacy would fall. Since we live in a world where emoji usage, alongside other digital signs, has become a kind of default mode of writing in everyday communications, the question of whether they can be deployed for educational purposes is clearly a key one. As such, it has led to various pedagogical studies, most of which present positive findings in this regard. Increasingly, the pedagogical utilization of emoji is showing up in different school subjects, from mathematics (Holton and Symons 2021) to English (King 2016). Most of the studies indicate that emoji influence the "student's impressions of credibility, immediacy, and liking," as Vareberg et al. (2022) aptly observe.

To reiterate, the main idea of adopting a semioliteracy framework is to impart academic literacy through the discourse and semiotic functions of emoji, thus making the study of literacy relevant to students who do not learn well within the traditional curricular parameters (Glass and Kang 2018). It also allows students to utilize the devices they bring to class in a constructive way. Studies such as the one by Wood et al. (2012) have shown, in fact, that excessive and distracting in-class cell phone usage is a problem across various institutions and learning environments (Mapes and Hea 2018). Giving verbal instructions as to how to complete an assignment or answer questions about the instructions tend to be ignored, because of the availability of mobile phone communications. This has often led to the need for remedial pedagogy – which itself has hardly ever turned out to be effective. So, the task set out by the Petcoff project was to envision how to incorporate mobile devices directly into the classroom, thus not going against the grain but rather inserting oneself pedagogically within it. The task was, however, complicated by the fact that the school system required procuring approved teaching tools; that is, tools that met the needs of both the individual (and challenged) student while being accessible and relatable to the adult learner demographic. The project found that the connecting link between the two sets of learners was emoji communication. It showed that the semioliteracy model was the most effective one because it allowed for the integrated use of discursive, presentational, and recursive aspects of literacy training. The approach is one potential response to the Conference on College Composition and Communication's (CCCC) 1974 Students' Right to Their Own Language declaration, which was intended to enact a strategy of inclusion of all students, including struggling ones.

The CCCC is a national professional association of college and university writing instructors in the United States. It was established in 1949 as an organization within the National Council of Teachers of English and continues to be one of the largest organizations dedicated to literacy research, theory, and teaching worldwide. A key aspect of CCCC-based research is to seek out teaching tools that are geared toward a diverse population of students, while avoiding instruction that would be perceived as demeaning or even just subpar with respect to the general student population. Given the common use of emoji as visual communicative signs, complementing verbal ones, the claim made here is that they can bridge the gap between student populations effectively, given their relevance to all types of learners (especially outside the classroom). Petcoff's goal was to bring emoji into the developmental (remedial) education classroom so that pedagogy could tap into how students used them to communicate, think, and create meaning on their own, outside of traditional literacy-based rules and conventions.

The term *developmental education* was used for the first time in 1970 by Frank Christ to describe the kinds of pedagogical efforts developed to teach students in his Learning Assistance Center (Arrendale 2014: 15–16). His idea was to assist students with learning difficulties, with special needs, or from underprivileged backgrounds to achieve expected competencies in core academic skills such as literacy and numeracy via pedagogy designed specifically for them. However, by the millennium, the typology of developmental students had become more complex, as the student population became more and more multiethnic and multiracial, differentiating itself from the primarily white population of the mid-1940s to the early 1970s, when, as Arrendale (2014: 19) notes, the developmental categories were enlarged to encompass "traditional white male students, nontraditional males and females, and federal legislative priority groups: first-generation college, economically-disadvantaged, and students of color," as well as older students returning to education or attending college for the first time. Today, this diversity of is no longer an exception, but a reality in all kinds of classroom situations. More recent scholarship has further expanded the typology (Hassel and Phillips 2022: 11), embracing any group of learners with the common need to improve the basic literacy skills that have been mastered by nondevelopmental peers.

Like the new literacy approach, semioliteracy pedagogy envisions all types of students as equal learners. In the current technological environment, notions of literacy are changing and adapting in response to the ways people communicate globally. A primary consequence of this reality is the need for what is now called "situated practice," which focuses on the connection between classroom learning and real-world experiences, building upon the concrete personal experiences of learners. Another consequence is the need for the critical framing of knowledge, whereby the sociocultural contexts in which a concept (in history, literature, science, mathematics, etc.) is developed is given prominence via semioliterate techniques. Finally, the crux for updating pedagogy is to adopt all kinds of sign systems as part of a semioliteracy approach. It is in turning theory into practice that emoji-based instruction comes concretely into play, since it allows for the student's emoji literacy to become an intrinsic part of learning other kinds of literacies. Emoji bring learner experiences, knowledge, and interests to the artificial classroom learning environment, allowing them to include their perspectives directly into the learning process. This activates Vygotsky's zone of proximal development, since the learners are immersed in taking part in something that is new or unfamiliar, but within the zone of their own life-worlds.

Semioliteracy teaching falls into the tradition called "authentic pedagogy," formulated in counter-position to "didactic pedagogy," traced back to the early twentieth century ideas of John Dewey in the United States and Maria Montessori in Italy (Kalantzis and Cope 2012: 95–117). The central notion is a focus on the learner's own experiences and talents, adopting materials that are relevant to their everyday lives. When it comes to reading and writing, authentic literacy pedagogy promotes internalized understanding rather than the abstract formalities of grammar and vocabulary. In the context of our increasingly diverse and globally interconnected lives, authentic literacy cannot be assigned only to developmental or specialized learning, since everyone is immersed in the same communicative reality. The traditional curricula operate on various rules of inclusion and exclusion, which involve a hierarchical ordering of literacy practices, often dismissing textual types such as picture books or popular fiction. In so doing, however, groups of learners are disenfranchised and may lose out on opportunities to achieve literacy practically.

In sum, semioliteracy transcends conventional print literacy pedagogy via the adoption of the different modes of communicating today. The use of emoji, which are part of a quasi-universal mode of communicating, allows for a form of situated learning that can potentially lead to the mastery of such literacies (as will be discussed). It moves away from the assembly line–based pedagogy of the past to a more personalized one that would unfold within the Vygotskian zones of proximal development, allowing the learners to progress at their own pace but within contextualized limits.

Applications to Healthcare Education

Semioliteracy is a notion that is best related to a "semiotic consciousness," whereby the different modes and media of sign use come into play in all forms of communication and understanding. It is also the basis for traditions and dialogical practices in medicine, given the connection among health, disease, and sign systems. In an age when specialized medical approaches to disease and health can no longer be isolated from the technological cultures and situations in which they occur, a goal of emoji-based practices and professional training in the public healthcare system is to enhance the ways of conveying to the general public the meaning of diseases through a visual communicative template. The Palaganas studies aiming to assess this approach are discussed in detail in Chapter 4. Suffice it to say here that this has practical implications for healthcare teams and the conduct of public health practices. The ancient Greek physician Hippocrates – the assumed founder of both medicine and semiotics – put it insightfully as follows: "It's far more important to know what person the disease has than what disease the person has" (cited in Adams 1849: 23).

Given their high emotivity, as discussed, one area in which emoji use is receiving particular attention is in physician–patient interactions. Renne et al. (2022) claim that it allows physicians and patients to better understand each other, making symptoms and clinically relevant information visible (literally). Dr. Shuhan He was actually a cocreator of the anatomical heart and the lung emoji introduced globally in 2020. He was also one of our interviewees for this book (as mentioned). The capacity of emoji visuality to convey meaning

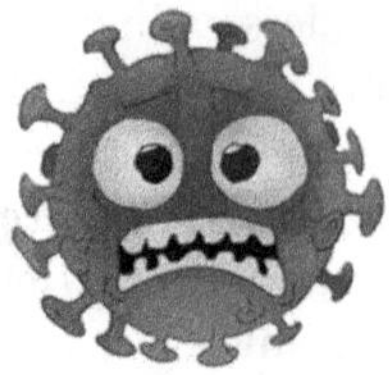

Figure 1.4 Coronavirus emoji

powerfully emerged during the coronavirus pandemic, when cartoonish emoji-like pictographs of the virus became Internet memes. An example can be seen in Figure 1.4.

The above (made-up) emoji (similar to those on the Internet) transmits in a comical way what the health enemy looked like. Aware of the emotive power of such images, Graphic Medicine, a health platform, adopted visuality systematically as a means to communicate with the general public, devising emoji, comics, and cartoons for informing or warning people about the effects of a disease (Tuohy 2018). Interestingly, the US-based Centers for Disease Control (CDC) hired medical illustrators to create a visible identity for the coronavirus that would draw attention to its danger via the power of iconic presence, perhaps inspired by the emoji used in this area of digital communications. Whether the emoji was actually effective or not during the height of the pandemic to get people to adopt prophylactic measures is a moot point – it became, as Sonnevend (2020: 461) remarks, "a key [source] for imagining the crisis."

Emoji rather than text are useful in public health messaging, especially when communicating in situations where multiple languages are involved. Moreover, they might be more effective stimuli for getting people to adopt healthy practices than admonitions via words. A study by Lotfinejad et al. (2020) found that emoji were useful in global health efforts to get people to wash their hands: "Concerning the infiltration of emojis into scientific literature, it is imperative to evaluate the impact of these symbols in health-related fields in order to harness their potential advantages for appropriate research applications and stave off scientific miscommunication." In situations other than public health messaging, what keeps doctors from using emoji with patients is that there is not a clear context or set of rules of etiquette for them – to be discussed in Chapters 3 and 5.

Epilogue

The fact that emoji have spread across the world is evidence that alphabet-based writing is no longer the exclusive mode. McLuhan (1964) had observed long before the Internet age that the capacity for daily global communications would create a sense of being caught permanently in the present, implying that there is an immediacy to such communications that makes them ephemeral. The print communications of the past were constructed in a way that impelled people to perceive a continuity between the present, the past, and the future, mirroring the chronology of events as laid out in, say, a novel or historical treatise. In the age of digital communications, we may have lost some of this sense, since communications are fragmented, reproduced constantly and renewed quickly. As a result, we feel suspended nowhere and everywhere, which, McLuhan asserted, is the same form of consciousness experienced by those who lived primarily in oral (and pictogram-using) cultures, whose sense of history and reality was more episodic than chronologically linear.

Emoji fall under this paradigm, where history is perceived more and more as a set of episodes than a concatenated linear set of events, much like the images in a picture book or a comic book. Although they surfaced as a means to enhance broader comprehension of written texts in the global village, culturally stylized forms have nonetheless emerged for various reasons (as we saw earlier). Recall the example of facial emoji. By and large, the creators of the smileys have attempted to make them as culturally neutral as possible. But, almost right after their introduction into common usage, new emoji were constructed that embedded culturally based meanings, either explicitly or unwittingly. The nerd 🤓 and sleuth 🕵 emoji, for example, require understanding what a "nerd" or "sleuth" implies in culture-specific ways. These would make absolutely no sense to, say, a society living outside the realm of modern urbanized popular cultures from which these signs emerged. It is perhaps more accurate to say that some emoji are higher on a "universality scale" than others. The slightly frowning 🙁, smiling 🙂, and face with rolling eyes 🙄 emoji can be located higher up on the scale; others, such as the robot face 🤖, are likely to have "mid-scale" comprehensibility; and others still, such as the live long and prosper emoji 🖖, are likely to have a lower-scale comprehensibility. The last emoji alludes to a pop culture referent – the 1960s *Star Trek* program on American network television, where it surfaced as the Vulcan peace sign. Although the sign has become somewhat of a common symbol in many parts of the world, its interpretation is constrained by various variables, such as the age of the emoji users and their geo-historical background. As such, emoji might represent a *langue* all its own, to use Saussure's (1916) term, and one that is constantly evolving, accruing subtle meanings known only to seasoned users. But it is a different kind of *langue* in that it has eliminated the traditional distinction between separate verbal and visual modes of representation and communication – that is, between verbality and visuality.

But it is exactly the emoji *langue*'s connection and relevance to the modern world that can play a key role in education at all levels. Emoji allow for a coordination of ideas expressed verbally and visually, and thus for a semioliterate organization that integrates visual characters and verbal ideas expressed cohesively, subject to cultural, subjective, and technological variance factors. Because emoji are structures that can be applied to any message on the spot, they are highly effective for allowing the activation of agency and alterity factors that are now practically de rigueur in the multicultural, multiracial, and developmentally differentiated classrooms for real learning to unfold. The dangers of overusing or misusing emoji is part of a broader pedagogical discussion that can be elaborated (Chapter 6); overall, there is little doubt that they can level the educational playing field for all students.

In sum, emoji have made hybrid literacy both a fact and an educational imperative. The argument will be made that such literacy is a point of departure for imparting academic literacy (Chapter 2) and a means for facilitating healthcare communications (Chapter 4) as well as the education of healthcare professionals (Chapter 5). In the print age, with its emphasis on linear progression, humanity constructed linear-narrative models of history that suggested that the future was infinitely far away and that personal and social evolution was involved in finding a path toward it; in the Internet age, there is no comparable cognitive linearity; there is mainly connectivity that makes us feel situated within a network structure.

So, as a final introductory thought about emoji, one can legitimately ask: Are emoji a revolution in human communication or a passing trend? Will they be around in, say, 2089? Emoji in themselves are not revolutionary, given that they retrieve pictographic forms of writing in a new technologically standardized way. So, they will likely morph into something else or disappear entirely as the technology changes. The Oxford Dictionary may have been right after all, sensing that emoji captured a moment in time. It could also well be that emoji bear an unconscious desire that reflects the times – the need to render communication as friendly as possible. In conducting interviews with students, on the part of all three authors of this book, the overall view that emoji convey a “sunny” tone to human interaction surfaced commonly. It is no accident that the most common emoji bear the color of the sun.

2 Emoji Literacy as a Teaching Tool

Prologue

The emergence of emoji literacy (as a component of hybrid literacy and of semioliteracy more generally) has been the topic of a plethora of studies since 2015, showing (overall) that emoji are part of an ever-broadening multimodal writing competence acquired through daily exposure and utilization on digital devices. In the previous chapter, some of the implications that this has had for the notion of literacy were broached in a generic way. In this chapter, we will look more specifically at the meaning and functions of emoji literacy in a specific educational setting, since these provide practical insights that can guide the overall objective of integrating emoji writing into all kinds of education-instructional paradigms. The chapter describes the main findings of a pilot project conducted by Omonpee Petcoff (one of the authors of this book), which was designed to assay the premise that emoji literacy can be used as a basis for imparting basic academic reading and writing literacy.

A primary psychological-semiotic feature of emoji is that they encompass a tripartite referentiality based on pictographic, ideographic, and logographic representations, which enlist different levels of meaning, from the concretely iconic and simulative, as can be seen in pictograms such as facial emoji, to the highly abstract modality that ideographic forms entail, whereby the image of, say, a heart, must be mapped against a connotative system of understanding that is symbolic and aesthetic at once. As such, the pedagogical incorporation of emoji as learning tools would allow students to gain intuitive access to what Umberto Eco (1974) called the "encyclopedia of knowledge" that sign forms encode – an unconscious system of shared knowledge that governs the production and interpretation of signs within specific contexts. Every semiotic act, such as the use of a smiley emoji, involves meaning elements that are embedded in that encyclopedia. Moreover, in hybrid writing a bimodal system of learning, verbal and visual, is activated, which has been found to optimize learning in different disciplines (Danesi 2015), and thus arguably would support the gaining of literacy in specific educational contexts. Verbal and visual forms of literacy involve two main differential processes – phonemic (which is discrete) and visual (which is holistic). A word written with alphabet characters is designed to represent its phonemic structure (to varying degrees). So, understanding it involves carrying out a mental assembly of its parts (alphabet characters standing for phonemes) to reconstruct through the assemblage the spoken word. On the other hand, emoji are pictorial signs that stand for referents in layered ways. Like a painting, the meaning of the emoji cannot be gleaned by assemblage of the parts to reconstruct a word; rather, it involves holistic processing, which produces an image schema in the mind of its meaning potential (discussed further in Chapter 3).

As discussed, emoji are not just projections of paralinguistic-prosodic features and bodily kinesics onto the screen, although they do encompass these functions in various ways when the content entails them. They are capsules of visual thought that influence how we process meaning in tandem with words. Emoji literacy raises a whole set of questions, such as what part of speech (if any) will an emoji assume? A cloud emoji is likely to be perceived as a noun corresponding to the word cloud. A sunrise emoji, on the other hand, showing the shape of a sun as it rises up from a background, suggests either the noun *sunrise* or the verb *rising* (of the sun). Now, these very same emoji forms could be used to describe some emotion, such as a cloudy mood or a sunny disposition, thus functioning as metaphorical forms. In effect, it is difficult to assign emoji to specific parts of speech, because they are conceptually multifunctional.

The main practical implication of harnessing emoji literacy is, beyond its bimodal efficacy as a learning tool, that it is an intrinsic part of a discourse of which students today are practitioners – that is, they are already emoji literate even before entering a classroom. The pedagogical question becomes: Can the psychological-semiotic elements of this literacy be extracted and transferred to the acquisition of a broader academic literacy? The goal of the Petcoff project was to address this question in a specific way, so as to assess the validity of semioliteracy as a framework for instruction in alignment with the needs of a diverse set of learners. The results of the project (Petcoff 2023) indicate that incorporating emoji literacy into literacy-training courses for developmental learners constitutes a highly effective instructional strategy capable of activating the modal flow of learning from visuality to verbality (discussed later in this chapter).

Subsequently, we will assess and discuss the more general use of emoji in education, at least at the present time, given the communication technologies used routinely (Chapter 6). The most relevant aspect of "emoji pedagogy," as it can be called, is that emoji are so readily understandable across languages and individuals, raising the possibility that they will fit easily into the ever-expanding paradigm of intercultural and intersubjective education. In contrast to strictly verbal language and writing scripts, emoji present content that is more readily shareable in all kinds of learning contexts, no matter what language is used in the educational process, and no matter what background the student takes to the learning context. It is the visual-holistic nature of these signs that can provide a conceptual basis on which to teach discrete-linear verbal forms of literacy via transference of notions gained visually to the same notions to be acquired verbally. It is the shift from visuality to verbality that makes emoji effective in promoting transference learning.

Emoji Literacy

In the previous chapter, we discussed various perspectives of what literacy implies and how it has evolved through the ages, from being conceived primarily as based on print, to current multimedia literacies, of which hybrid literacy – a blend of emoji and verbal text – is the most common form. Overall, the different literacies can be categorized under the rubric of semioliteracy (the ability to use and coordinate signs in different media forms, verbal and nonverbal). The objective here is to focus on emoji literacy itself, so as to map it against other literacies and to assay its pedagogical utility. As Marissa King (2016) notes, the utility comes from the fact that "students seamlessly navigate emoji usage [in a way that] is similar to the critical reading skills we practice in class." She also envisions a practical aspect of emoji in a classroom environment whereby students can themselves create guides for new emoji users, including teachers, thus impelling them to focus on how emoji generate meaning and how to constrain or refine meaning according to context – which is a primary goal of traditional literacy pedagogy. As the Petcoff project described here showed, in fact, teachers do not need to be emoji experts to use them, since they too can enlist students to explicate to them, thus constituting in itself a valuable student-centered pedagogical activity. And because emoji use is constantly evolving, knowledge gaps can be filled in by the students who are knowledgeable of changes in emoji modalities, which they can discuss in terms of their evolving discourse-semiotic functions in class. King (2016) concludes as follows:

> Welcoming emojis into the classroom is one way to use student experience to develop school skills. Rather than detract from learning goals, our students' rich social media lives can contribute to deeper learning. By connecting to skills our students already use online, perhaps we can make school seem even more relevant.

New forms of literacy are cropping up because of the Internet and mobile technology innovations, where virtual communities have emerged, and can no longer be excluded from the classroom. The term *literacy* today thus encompasses a broad range of meaning, including traditional literacy, digital literacy, media literacy, computer literacy, and information literacy, among many others, which are all part of a generic semioliteracy, defined as the ability to use and comprehend the different sign forms and textual structures available in different media (mentioned earlier). Take, for instance, the type of literacy required to engage in Twitter (now called X) communities, typically called *twitteracy*. In a relevant study, Greenhow and Gleason (2012) explored tweeting as a literacy practice, finding that it combined traditional and digital modes of writing (modes that involve abbreviation, acronymy, alphanumeracy, etc.), impacting both informal and formal registers. Black (2008) had already called this "global literacy," because it cuts across political and cultural borders, with its incorporation of common cultural artifacts, as well as multimodal pastiches of text, image, and sound. Davies (2012) found that self-presentation and friendship management were the primary concerns of social media users. The photos on Twitter and the emoji used strategically allowed online interlocutors to construct "pictorial bio-narratives" of themselves on which friends could comment, add nuance, or generate tags and hashtags as conduits of subsequent interaction. Authorship of a tweet is now neither individualistic nor completely original, because remixing is fundamental to how people create these texts.

Most tweets are conversational in style and function – exchanges between friends, associates, colleagues, and acquaintances. Information exchange is not the main attraction of Twitter – indeed, only a small percentage of tweets can be considered to be information-based. Some have designated Twitter as a venue for "social grooming," that is, for presenting oneself in a favorable way to others in order to gain attention and to gather followers. It is also used to promote one's personal agenda and views. Institutions of various kinds now use Twitter as a source of contact with clients and colleagues. The limited length of each tweet, the desire for attracting followers, and the constant flow of tweets are all part of twitteracy.

The new literacies have attenuated (and even eliminated in some cases) the traditional boundaries between categories such as authorship, readership, production, and consumption (Gee 1996, Kress 2003). Bryden et al. (2013) found that tweeting constitutes a new kind of discourse code with its own symbolic artifacts, such as hashtags. It requires knowing how to self-present oneself to the Twitter community, participate in it (*mentions*), distribute information (*retweets*), and organize conversations (*hashtags*). Based on how digital signs and the traditional types of literacy signs are now used in tandem, Haas and Takayoshi (2011) have introduced a useful distinction between "standard literacies," which are characteristic of formal offline contexts, and online "everyday literacies," which entail knowledge of the new digital signs, including emoji. The two are dynamically intertwined, leading to a new form of diglossia. They may also complement each other in covert ways. Barden (2012) noticed an increase in standard literacy competence in dyslexic middle school subjects, after they had engaged with multimodal digital text structures. This led the subjects to a better understanding of sequence and semiotic relation in linear texts. In other words, their everyday literacy was enhanced via engagement with online everyday literacy.

In schools, it is not uncommon today for educators and students to move back and forth between online and offline literacies depending on writing task and function (Crystal 2011). Arguably, digital writing practices may have increased sensitivity to writing itself, producing a kind of expanded semioliteracy competence, which involves, in the case of hybrid literacy (emoji-with-text):

(1) knowing when and how to use emoji versus verbal script;
(2) knowing how to communicate meaning according to mode (visual or verbal) in terms of specific content;
(3) recognizing discourse and semiotic differences between print and emoji literacies;
(4) understanding how traditional literacy can be enhanced with digital writing via multimodality (not only emoji, but photos, videos, and audio);
(5) knowing how to communicate in virtual spaces according to online community;
(6) knowing how different styles and registers now interact in online and offline contexts;
(7) knowing how to mine information from the Internet and use it for both online and offline communications.

The study of the different literacies that have emerged is sometimes included under the general rubric of digital literacy (Gilster 1998; Hobbs 2017). This can be defined as the ability to decipher, create, understand, and interpret digital signs and texts correctly or meaningfully. Many features of digital literacy parallel face-to-face communication. The term used in reference to this is "digital orality," which implies that today's digital media are retrieving a form of orality that is simulated in how the written word is now laid out and formed – namely, as a visual episodic form of recording ideas and relevant narratives, recalling in an indirect way the hieroglyphic writing used to record episodes and events relevant to Egyptian society and history. Like oral societies of the past, digital communications now typically entail real-time responses, whereas traditional written communications involve a time lag in receiving responses. As Walter Ong argued in *Orality and Literacy* (1982), the orality mode of early cultures can be called "primary," while the orality that has surfaced through electronic communications can thus be called "secondary." So, paradoxically, when we communicate by writing (emails, text messages, tweets, and so on), our expectations from the act of communication are similar to those of oral communication – that is, we expect an immediate or quasi-immediate response and a style of writing that simulates oral expression. The central features of secondary orality are as follows:

(1) It is elliptical and compressed in ways that parallel oral speech.
(2) It is mainly synchronous (occurring in real time) like vocal speech, while it is also editable, like writing.
(3) It is typically informal and highly conversational in style and mode of delivery.
(4) It encourages immediate replies from one's interlocutor, as in oral communication.

Emoji fit in perfectly with such evolving forms of digital communication. Their sophisticated semiotic modalities, ranging from iconicity to symbolism, can be adopted and adapted to impart an integrated competence in relevant discursive, presentational, and recursive functions, thereby making them an effective teaching tool. Although emoji meanings may vary cross-culturally, across platforms, and intersubjectively, they nonetheless present themselves as part of a largely recognizable pictographic language that is "spoken" (as a secondary oral mode) by people throughout the world. As such it is inherently a democratic language that makes little or no distinction as to the class or background of interlocutors. The 1974 CCCC Students' Right to Their Own Language declaration (Chapter 1) prophetically envisaged that a digital literacy, such as the emoji one, was required to highlight the importance of student rights. Below is the original declaration (Perryman-Clark et al. 2015: 22):

> We affirm the students' right to their own patterns and varieties of language – the dialects of their nurture or whatever dialects in which they find their own identity and style. Language scholars long ago denied that the myth of a standard American dialect has any validity. The claim that any one dialect is unacceptable amounts to an attempt of one social group to exert its dominance over another. Such a claim leads to false advice for speakers and writers, and immoral advice for humans. A nation proud of its heritage and its cultural and racial variety will preserve its heritage of dialects. We affirm strongly that teachers must have the experiences and training that will enable them to respect diversity and uphold the right of students to their own language.

The goal is to teach academic discourse through the personal discourse(s) of students: "We should structure and select materials geared to complex reading problems and oriented to the experience and sophistication of our students" (Perryman-Clark et al. 2015: 22). Exploring how emoji literacy qualifies as a shared discourse and thus a common language across groups of students and how it can be used to impart academic literacy is a concrete response to the CCCC's overall objectives. Recalling Arnheim (1969), the main semiotic premise for adopting emoji literacy as a teaching tool is that it activates mechanisms of visuality, located in the right hemisphere of the brain, as a means to co-activate the verbal mechanisms in the left hemisphere.

This is nothing new to educators – it is simply an update. Pictures and diagrams as have always constituted a repertoire of "visual tools" for teachers in all disciplines. In all such devices, shape, combination, and reference are intertwined, much like verbality: "👁 ❤ U" is not the same as "U ❤ 👁"; and 😁 is not the same as 😵. This interplay on form, structure, and content is at the core of meaning-making in semioliterate teaching.

A Mixed Methodology Emoji Study

To examine the instructional viability of using emoji to impart academic literacy to students struggling with reading and writing, Petcoff conducted a comprehensive study in the spring of 2019, ending in the spring of 2023, using various methods and instructional tools. Prior to what would become the study in question, Petcoff conducted a pilot study in which thirty-nine developmental first-year students in a Texas community college enrolled in three sections during one semester participated in the experiment. Of that number, only seventeen responses proved to be usable. The students reflected a diverse learning population. Then, to obtain more definitive data, Petcoff refined her methods and tools. In the revised study, sixty-eight samples were submitted, with forty-six deemed usable. She also synthesized the number of research questions from five to three as well as the focus of the study. The new project aimed to chronicle and analyze the results of using both traditional writing forms and emoji with the students in view of achieving state-mandated literacy levels. While the project was based on a specific population, it bears broader implications (which will be discussed in subsequent chapters). An impetus for the study was that Petcoff, a Developmental Education Reading and Writing instructor at a Texas community college, became dismayed with students' incessant texting during classes. No matter what was being taught and how many times the students were asked to not use cellphones during a lesson, they were seemingly transfixed by their mobile devices and rarely abandoned them to give their attention to classroom procedures and content. So, the questions that she asked herself can be paraphrased as follows: Why not use their phone literacy profitably in the classroom? How can the emoji literacy that this entails be employed practically to teach academic literacy?

In 2018, the Texas Higher Education Coordinating Board passed House Bill 2223, which mandated that community colleges would no longer offer different levels of developmental reading and writing instruction. This was due in large part to concerns about student retention and graduation rates. So, it was decided that students should no longer be required to take developmental courses prior to enrolling in their respective degree programs. Under the bill, a college could offer one adult basic education remedial course, for all developmental reading and writing students with varying degrees of literacy levels, including those whose first language was not English, students with cognitive disabilities, and other challenged learners. The course was to be taken as a corequisite with a first-year reading or writing-intensive credit course. As part of the Texas Success Initiative Assessment (TSIA), it was expected that developmental education teachers help challenged students acquire the necessary skills to be able to manage college-level education – an unrealistic objective given that the relevant preparatory course lasted eight weeks and was taken simultaneously with college-level writing courses, with few (if any) relevant pedagogical resources.

In open-access learning institutions, pedagogical needs are defined by mandatory entrance assessments. Teaching materials in such cases are limited, which conveys the impression that open-access instruction is less important than its four-year counterparts (Hassel and Phillips 2022). Only a handful of publishers have attempted to fill the void; so, commonly, developmental reading and writing instructors will typically have to prepare their own pedagogical materials. It is within this situational latitude that the project was conducted, using emoji as a primary tool for imparting the mandated literacy levels, taking advantage of the mobile-device literacy that students brought to the classroom, which they grasped concretely.

Method

Three specific research questions (RQ) guided the study.

- RQ1: Which TSIA reading content area skills can be improved by using emoji to teach literacy?
- RQ2: Which corresponding writing TSIA content area skills can be improved by using emoji?
- RQ3: How do the discursive properties of emoji aid in developmental reading and writing literacy improvement?

To address RQ1 and RQ2, a Google Forms survey, *Reading and Writing with Emoji* (*QE*), was used in which participants could employ emoji, textisms (SMSes), and traditional writing styles to answer questions that measured their mastery of various TSIA skills. The list of questions is found in Petcoff (2023). A thirty-six-question survey was developed from this and administered in week eight of the sixteen-week semester. The students had received preliminary instruction in all content areas and the survey selected was based on their demonstrable level of mastery. For RQ3, a level of shared emoji competence (discursive and semiotic) was assessed via an analysis of the survey responses. The survey comprised both multiple choice and short answer questions, providing data on five main themes:

Section 1: Summarizing with Traditional Writing versus Emoji Textisms

This involved grasping the role that emoji play in the minds of the participants. The students were asked to watch a TedTalk by linguist John McWhorter titled *Txting is Killing Language, JK!!!*, which was used to introduce them to current scholarship on textspeak and emoji, given that it explores opposing viewpoints on their use. On the basis of the video, students were then instructed to write a "basic paragraph" on the video, using traditional (academic) writing. They had received some training previously in how to summarize and paraphrase a text, in line with the benchmarks set by the Texas Success Initiative (TSI) Reading and Writing Assessment categories – the TSI is a legislatively mandated program designed to guide Texas public institutions of higher education in helping determine whether entering, nonexempt students are ready for entry-level college coursework in the areas of English Language Arts Reading and mathematics:

Reading (Comprehension) Skills

- Knowing how to extract the main idea from the text and to identify its supporting details
- Ability to perceive how language was used by the maker of the text (in this case a video presenter)
- Ability to draw inferences from the text
- Knowing how to enlist basic literary analysis to understanding a text

Writing (Production)

- Ability to control sentence structure to deliver meaning
- Awareness of how to put the parts of the text into conceptual-structural agreement, so that they cohere together thematically
- Grasping the overall sentence logic involved, including the appropriate style used
- Knowing how to revise (edit) the writing

The assessment of the responses was based on how the participants were able to display the basic paragraph writing skills in conjunction with proficiency levels in summarizing and paraphrasing content as defined by the TSI.

Section 2: Interpreting Emoji-Textism Writing

This aimed to determine how the participants utilized emoji as part of visual literacy. Specifically, they were asked to summarize the previously written basic paragraph using only textspeak (texting abbreviations and emoji). In this task, students were encouraged to pretend they were texting a friend about the McWhorter video. They were then instructed to take screen shots of their writing and upload them to a designated survey portal on the school's Blackboard. This part of the project was intended to assay how the participants analyzed and reflected on the blending of emoji writing, textese (the use of textisms), and traditional writing. The participants were asked whether they found the task of summarizing the TedTalk via traditional text or with textese and emoji easier or harder. As a follow-up, the students were asked to assess which method of writing provided them with the optimal means for conveying the most information and relevant reflections. As per the TSI, an appropriate analysis of a written text through writing is one of the criteria used to denote mastery of integrated reading and writing skills. More specifically, this part of the project sought to ascertain if and to what extent emoji could be used to teach and improve literacy skills in developmental reading and writing students.

Section 3: Efficacy of Emoji versus Traditional Writing

Developmental reading and writing classrooms are comprised of students with varying degrees of English language proficiency; therefore, the instructional tools must be crafted to address the needs and cognitive styles of the students. Traditional literacy instructional tools involving alphabetic literacy were employed as well to assess proficiency levels, varying according to a student's ability to carry out basic reading and writing skills such as decoding and encoding written texts, sounding out phonemes, and mastering sentence structure (Albright and Luke 2012). While these skills are certainly important, the traditional forms of instruction do not allow learners whose first language is not English or developmental learners to grasp such skills, without some specific type of aid by the teacher. To circumvent this dilemma, educators have normally turned to various options, such as visual literacy pedagogy to create a level of learning within the learning challenged classroom, which is similar to the storybook-phonics approach used to teach reading literacy to children. While exposure to spoken language in childhood does not require any intervention on the part of adults, since children construct the language on their own without training, learning how to read and write requires such intervention. One way to do so is to associate written words with images, and even individual letters as constituents of visual referents – an approach known as *phonics*, introduced in the nineteenth century. One of the first examples of a phonics reader is the 1836 one by American educator William Holmes McGuffey, which shows pictures for words, allowing the reader to match picture, word, and its spelling conjointly.

A key study by Taylor et al. (2017) compared teaching with visual phonics to teaching how to read in other ways, concluding that it was more effective in languages that are based on the alphabet principle. All forms of writing mediate our sense of reality. McLuhan's (1962) basic premise was that a new writing medium, such as alphabetic writing, rewires the brain, orienting it toward its specific features (linearity, sequence of ideas, abstraction, etc.). In alphabetic writing, the abstraction layer is, in effect, a mediating one. This means that the brain does not "see" a referent directly through some picture form, but rather must extrapolate the referent via the "mental phonics" of the word. So, when we read a word such as *cat*, we must decipher the phonics of the word first and then extrapolate the referent from it (as mentioned earlier). Visual literacy teaching is designed to broach the gap between visualizing a referent and reconstructing it via phonic abstraction.

Sections 4 and 5: Emoji Semantics and Pragmatics

These sections involved questions related to the semantic and pragmatic aspects of emoji usage, such as the ability to aptly choose between two or more similar emoji to complete a phrase. They could thus measure and assess the students' fluency in emoji use as a discourse code and their ability to code-switch between emoji/textese and alphabetic literacy according to the TSI categories.

Locations and Data Collection

Students received invitations to take the survey via a QR code on fliers. Interested participants accessed the Google Forms survey and completed the Informed Consent Page prior to beginning the study. They were directed to use their cellphones or other mobile devices; they were also allowed to use the emoji keyboard on a computer. Table 2.1 displays each RQ along with the corresponding evidence for addressing each one and the methodologies employed to analyze the data (note: INRW refers to a course designation).

Among the theoretical notions adopted for the analysis, Peircean and Jakobsonian ones were used as central ones. Charles Peirce (1938–58) put forth a triadic model of the sign, consisting of the physical sign itself (which he called the *representamen*), the referent that it encodes (the *object*), and the interpretation that the sign elicits or reveals (the *interpretant*). He called the dynamic interaction between the three parts *semiosis*, which can be defined as the making and interpreting of the meanings of signs. The *interpretant* is critical in guiding how signs are used and understood. In western culture, for instance, a cat is considered to be a domestic companion, among other cultural interpretants; in others, it is viewed instead as a sacred animal (akin to a sacred cow); and in others still it is considered to be a killer of rodents. Thus, while different words for cat might *refer* to virtually the same physical mammal in

Table 2.1 *Research questions*

Research question	Evidence collected to answer the question	Analysis of the evidence (approach/method)
RQ1: Which TSIA reading content area skills may be improved by using emoji to teach literacy?	Answers to survey questions based on the following TSIA reading content areas: • Main idea and supporting details • Inferences/vocabulary in context • Author's use of language	**Methodology 1:** Create a grading rubric for Section 1. The rubric will be based on reading and writing skills previously covered in class. Open code via Voyant-Tools (RQ1 and RQ2) **Methodology 2:** Create a multiple-choice answer key for Section 4 Assess/grade the section for correct answers (RQ1 and RQ2) Just like with classroom instruction, a combined reading and writing score of 70% will serve as mastery and/or improvement. A rubric outlining the content areas and defining mastery will be created
RQ2: Which writing TSIA content area skills may be improved by using emoji to teach literacy?	Answers to survey questions based on the following TSIA writing content areas: • Agreement • Sentence structure • Sentence logic	**Methodology 3:** Context sensitive text analysis (Huckin 1992) This methodology includes:
RQ3: How do emoji's recursive and discursive properties aid in literacy instruction?	Answers to all-emoji-based survey responses and explanations of emoji choice	(1) **Selecting an initial corpus** (the survey responses) (2) **Identifying salient patterns** (exploring emoji choice for words; Peircean semiotic relations; Jakobsonian language functions; sentence structure; grammar) (3) **Determining emoji word choice rationale** (assessing emoji use, choice, and level of literacy effectively conveyed and accurately comprehended) (4) **Selecting a study corpus** (using the INRW 0399 as my control group and measuring its success against INRW 0090 students) (5) **Verifying a pattern** (open coding both emoji and common words and phrases in responses) (6) **Developing a functional-rhetorical pattern** (determining emoji's recursive, discursive, and shared meaning-making efficacies) (RQ1, RQ2, and RQ3)

Table 2.2 *Research questions mapped against Google survey questions*

Research questions with survey questions groupings		
RQ1 and RQ2 overview		
RQ1: Which reading TSIA content area skills may be improved by using emoji to teach literacy?	**Evidence**: Answers to survey questions based on the following TSIA reading content areas:	
	TSIA reading content areas	**Survey questions**
	• Main idea and supporting details • Author's use of language	• Question 1: Traditional writing summary (Q1) • Question 2: Emoji-textism writing summary (Q2)
RQ2: Which writing TSIA content area skills may be improved by using emoji to teach literacy?	**Evidence**: Answers to survey questions based on the following TSIA writing content areas:	
	TSIA writing content areas	**Survey questions**
	• Agreement • Sentence structure • Sentence logic • Inferences	• Question 1 (Q1) • Question 2 (Q2) • Questions 19–26 (Q19–26)
RQ3 overview		
RQ3: How do emoji's recursive and discursive properties aid in literacy instruction?	**Evidence**: Answers to emoji-based survey responses and explanations of emoji choice. **Survey questions** • Questions 5–12: Interpreting emoji textisms (Q5–12) • Questions 19–26: Emoji as semantics and pragmatics, part one (Q19–26) • Questions 27–36: Emoji as semantics and pragmatics, part two (Q27–36) • Question 2: Emoji-textism summary paragraph (Q2) • Questions 3 and 4 (Q3 and Q4)	

different cultures (no matter what name is used), the *interpretant* of the words varies considerably, constituting the source of differential semiosis. In emoji use, this notion has great utility for describing individual and group differences in meaning-extraction. Jakobson (1960), as discussed in Chapter 1, provided a comprehensive model of communication, in which the emotive, conative, and phatic functions stand out as particularly useful in discussing emoji use.

The mapping of the RQs with Google's Survey Question groupings (a total of three) is shown in Table 2.2.

Findings

The project produced a highly detailed and sophisticated set of insights into how emoji are used proficiently by students to enhance their learning of literacy features. A complete analysis is found in Petcoff (2023). For the purposes of this book, only the main findings are considered, since these have implications for education more generally, as will be deliberated in subsequent chapters. The main findings are summarized as follows:

(1) **RQ1 results:** The reading TSIA skills improved considerably (when matched against the literacy levels brought originally by the students to the classroom), indicating that the use of emoji as a literacy instruction tool is a promising one, especially with regard to the TSIA categories of main idea, author's use of language, agreement, and inferences in a text or texts.
(2) **RQ2 results:** The TSIA writing skills also improved considerably: sentence structure, agreement, and sentence logic.
(3) **RQ3 results:** The results showed how the students were able to utilize the recursive and discursive properties of emoji, proficiently transferring them unconsciously to general literacy competence. They also showed how developmental literacy learners are able to access these properties via their shared understanding of emoji and texting as semiotic tools for constructing meaning.

RQ1 and RQ2 Results

The McWhorter video allowed for an assessment of RQ1 and RQ2, since it produced a variety of successful content-based summaries on the basic paragraph format. In the video there were several salient themes: 1. the emergence of emoji as a new form of writing; 2. the nature of emoji as an emergent communicative code; 3. negative views of emoji as causing the demise of traditional writing and reading; 4. texting as a new form of digital communication; and 5. texting as a new writing technology. At the heart of RQ1 and RQ2 findings are responses to survey questions 1 and 2. Q1 and Q2 assessed participants' abilities to view the McWhorter video as a visual text and to apply learned literacy skills to extrapolate key information from it, with Q1 requiring traditional writing responses and Q2 soliciting the same level of literacy skill mastery but with emoji-text hybrid writing.

The Q1 and Q2 responses were coded, and recurring words or phrases were categorized accordingly. The words *language* and *texting* were used the most, predictably, given the topic of the video. Most participants also wrote about McWhorter's assertions that texting has changed communication for the better and that people must adapt to this new method of communicating. A few participants wrote about emoji and textese as novel types of literacy; many resonated with McWhorter's claim that these constitute, in fact, a new writing competence that involves fewer formalities (punctuation, for example), which is not "killing" language, as many people seem to hold (according to

McWhorter). The results of the coding show that in the forty-six accepted submissions, all extrapolated the relevant main ideas from the video, presenting them in traditional writing (with some incorporation of new forms) via the basic paragraph format (Q1). Then, in Q2, students were asked to replicate the same amount of information but in an imaginary text to a friend and to use emoji hybrid writing. Character limits were not set, so that participants presented screenshots of texts of varying lengths. An example of a Q2 response appears below:

G14: John McWhorter, a professional linguist, decided to 🗣 on the relationship that language has with other ☁, societal, and political customs, titling his Ted Talk, "Txtng is killing language. JK!!!" First, McWhorter takes the time to express that the (cultural) way in which we communicate through 🔢 and in general (when "unmonitored"), has an impact on our mannerisms such as "speaking in word packets of maybe seven to 10 words" when with friends. Moreover, the speaker points out that as ⏱ passes, we feel certain statements that are now being said have gone 🙆 🚺 because were so used to the 📓 norms and that there is an emergent complexity in speech and society nowadays. Lastly, McWhorter proceeds to talk about how people from an earlier era (involved in politics) would have had a difficult time understanding slang because the young people of today developed a new language. In conclusion, language has a relationship with other 💃, societal, and political customs that are that are imperative to 💭 about.

Interestingly, the students used emoji to convey not only summary information, but also to show how they felt about either the subject matter or the task: The emotive emoji 😂 and 😆 were among the most commonly used ones for this purpose. This is significant because it implies that participants felt comfortable enough with emoji to use them to convey something that would not seem proper to do so in traditional writing: emotional state of mind or mood at the time of writing. Within the parameters of the study, therefore, emoji transcended a purely summary function, serving as well to convey how the writer was affected by the subject matter. Table 2.3 shows a chart summary of the most used emoji in survey question 2 vis-à-vis RQ1 and RQ2:

With regard to Q3 and Q4, the findings showed that all participants had the ability to recognize and convey the main differences between summarizing the video with traditional versus the hybrid form of writing. In reviewing all responses a pattern emerged: All but three of the participants indicated that writing in hybrid style (Q3) was easier, and all but one conceded that traditional writing was more appropriate in conveying content (RQ2). In terms of Q4 (semantic proficiency), the participants who found emoji easier to use indicated that this was so because they were more familiar with texting than they were with traditional academic writing. This familiarity resulted in a higher level of confidence in their ability to communicate effectively. Some even indicated that they developed their own slang within the hybrid code. They also found composing with the code easier because it does not impose rules

Table 2.3 *Research question 2 responses*

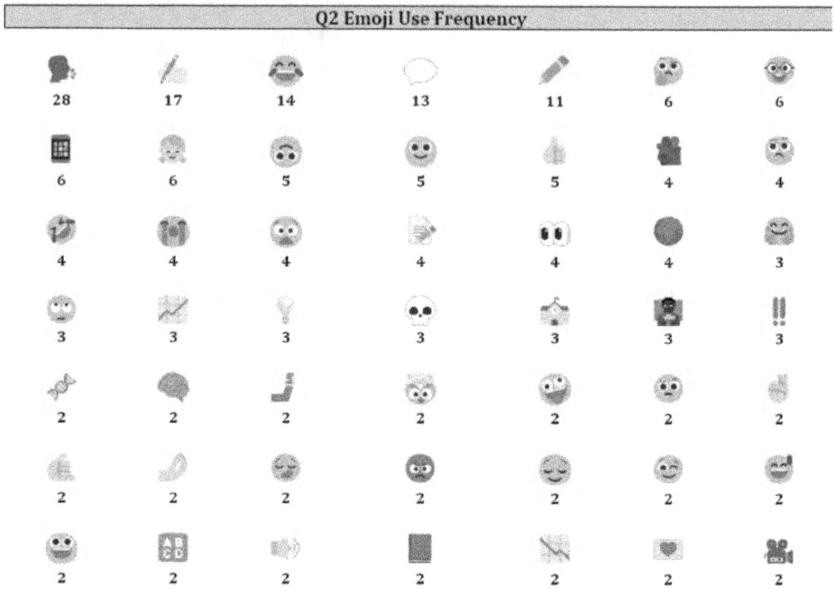

of punctuation and grammar associated with traditional writing. In spite of the ease associated with the hybrid code, significantly, most participants reported that they were able to convey more information via traditional writing. They cited lack of adequate emoji and textese choices for precise language representation, which they realized were needed to convey information within the basic paragraph format.

RQ3 Results

While RQ1 and RQ2 attempt to assess whether literacy can be mastered with emoji, RQ3's aim is to form a hypothesis as to how such mastery is achieved vis-à-vis a shared meaning or literacy consciousness. To answer RQ3, qualitative and quantitative methods were used to compare textese and emoji word choices with respect to the information presented via survey questions assessing each of the aforementioned literacy skills. From this, it was possible to identify which emoji are recurring ones, and how they matched the content appropriately. Interestingly, facial emoji were used as annotations to the views, while others were used them to summarize these in visual episodic ways. As expected, however, even with a shared emoji literacy, the participants did not demonstrate the same level or pattern of summarization and paraphrasing for

RQ2, especially in comparison to the traditional summary. In the hybrid compositions, the participants failed to address several main ideas present in the video presentation. This indicates that, while participants are familiar with textese and emoji, they might not be as useful when attempting to describe topics of an academic nature, at least entirely.

An analysis of the compositions also confirmed several hypotheses associated with semioliteracy instruction, including that fact that the students were able to code-switch between discursive and presentational aspects of meaning presentation (between verbal and emoji literacy) as well as able to use emoji recursively to strengthen meaning intent. The pictographic, ideographic, and logographic modalities also appeared to guide the selection of the emoji – for example, pictograms of the face added personal annotation, while emoji such as the fire and ghost emoji, which had ideographic abstract functions, were used in locations that required abstract conveyances of meaning. The findings also aligned with Borgman and McArdle's (2019) premise that any form of instruction that is tailored to be personable and accessible is highly effective in transferring content unconsciously (Borgman and McArdle 2019). This was enhanced by the fact that Google was used – a familiar and popular platform – and that hybrid writing was incorporated into the instructional process, creating conditions for congenial interactivity that make students feel at ease in participating (Tham 2018: 50).

From a Peircean perspective, the study highlighted the importance of the interpretant in sign use and comprehension – that is, of the variable element in meaning that involves the subjectivity of the learners. A sign, such as a facial emoji, generated a "dynamical interpretant," the actual semiotic reaction produced by the sign. This process is a continuous one of semiosis that progresses toward a "final interpretant," which is the result of the sign's effects on the mind. The process of semiosis, from dynamical to final interpretant, was seen when the students edited their compositions in stylized ways. The study also showed that the Vygotskian zone of proximal development theory, which allows students ample space to learn at their own pace, had a pragmatic effect, since it allowed students to learn within their own capacities.

Discussion

A significant overall finding of the Petcoff study was that the participants used emoji as a basis for comparing emoji literacy with traditional literacy, showing an awareness of the differences that they did not have beforehand. The level of detail in the student responses demonstrates a mastery of critical thinking about writing itself, and thus the crystallization of a metacognitive ability to reflect on their own thought processes and their relation to writing styles. What the project did not fully address, however, was identifying in specific psychological terms how the struggling student gleans or conveys meaning via emoji and how the discursive and presentational qualities of the emoji code influence the students' command of readability and writability. Some of the implications will be discussed in subsequent chapters.

While the study was based on a relatively small sample size, nonetheless, there is no reason to assume that similar findings would not emerge in other situations, and that the same psychological patterns would not apply. One area that needs further exploration is how the emoji code reflects an ever-expanding secondary orality (Chapter 1) and how this might affect print literacy utilization in an increasingly multimodal and multimedia classroom. One potential problem with semioliteracy instruction is the assumption that the learner has unconscious knowledge of semiotic modalities that the instructional process is designed to bring to the surface of consciousness. This was an assumption that seemed to have been confirmed, although not in any specific way.

Certainly, the most relevant finding was that emoji served as a means of imparting literacy awareness. As Lebduska (2014) has emphasized, the emoji phenomenon has contributed to a reconsideration of literacy and, thus, to an awareness-raising about the importance of reading and writing in a multimedia world. As she notes: "Emojis expand expression and in doing so open themselves to re-appropriation, interpretation and even misinterpretation, along with the affirming possibilities of artistic creation" (Lebduska 2014). In other words, emoji can supplement traditional literacies as well as unveiling new expressive potentials associated typically with visual art. It also implies the ability to locate signs and assemble them in ways that produce meanings in a specific context. As Gee (2003: 4) puts it:

> To understand or produce any word, symbol, image, or artifact in a given semiotic domain, a person must be able to situate the meaning of that word, symbol, image, or artifact within embodied experiences of action, interaction, or dialogue about that domain.

Two other findings were: (1) the participants mastered the TSIA reading and writing requirements, as the data collected for RQ1 and RQ2 demonstrated, and (2) there was a 70 percent shared meaning agreement for RQ3. These results correlated with the fact that the students formed an affinity group that allowed for consensus of emoji meaning and use across all data sets and levels. The implication from such findings is that emoji use in the classroom appears to provide an effective pedagogical strategy for imparting literacy to developmental students. But it also bears more general implications for education in today's global village (Chapter 6). As Lebduska (2014) quips: "At the end of the day, emojis are just as much a reflection of their creators as words, with just as much potential to express, explore, kvetch, and ultimately connect us to others. Though in some instances they supplant words entirely, they also open up new vistas of exchange and creativity." Among the more general implications that the study bears, the following can be mentioned at this point:

(1) Emoji appear to stimulate creative thinking, helping students (especially those with some background disadvantage) unpack hidden information in learning tasks.
(2) They motivate such students to explore new notions on their own, in terms of their unconscious emoji literacy, which can then be transferred to more academic forms of literacy.
(3) Most emoji reflect content that is easily understandable, no matter what the student's cultural, psychological, and sociological background, which makes them useful as classroom devices. While variation of meaning is present in any and all emoji use, arguably it is less expansive than it is with verbal communication. The fact that the same emoji (such as the smiley) is used by speakers of different languages, changing only in the interpretant in a few countries, is evidence that this premise is a plausible one. Being mindful of semiotic variance, actually, opens up the pedagogical process to relevant discussions that can be used to inform the meaning of literacy itself.
(4) Emoji can be tailored to reinforce specific learning objectives.
(5) They promote critical and creative thinking, which is transferable across subjects in school.
(6) When combined with other didactic materials, they complement the learning process in a supportive way.
(7) They can be adapted profitably for the enhancement of learning because they tap into patterns in contemporary culture.

Whatever the truth about the impact of emoji and other digital signs on traditional literacy systems, in an educational context, these are highly useful because they serve specific learning objectives, providing a contemporary vehicle for gaining the participation and collaboration of learners. In a related area, research by Angotti and Bayo (2012) found that video games in mathematics teaching engaged both students and teachers in a common effort to deliver content and develop mathematics skills. Similar research across disciplines, which was reviewed comprehensively by Malykhina (2014), corroborates the general principle that new devices are useful in education because they tap into cultural tendencies. Overall, therefore, emoji (like video games) seem to involve the following pedagogical effects:

(1) Students become more actively involved in learning tasks.
(2) When combined with other activities and with instruction from a teacher, they strengthen learning and foster motivation.
(3) They are relevant to the classroom today, since they are used widely in society generally.

(4) They allow students to explore different ways of writing and thinking.
(5) Beyond teaching, emoji and video games can also offer relevant information about how well a student is learning, because they can provide instantaneous feedback.

There are some issues or caveats that can be raised here. The main one can be articulated as follows: "What happens when emoji are replaced with some new interactive technology?" Of course, one could ask the same question about learning through print-based teaching materials that quickly went out of date. Through the utilization of hybrid learning materials and techniques (emoji-and-print learning blended together) the process is aligned with the knowledge that students already have. This may not extend to the future and thus to the ever-changing systems of communication. But all that can be said is that, with the present technology, the hybrid learning system is clearly an apt one to incorporate into the classroom. One can no longer expect a fairly homogenous background on the part of the students today. So, a raison d'être for a more integrated use of emoji literacy in today's classrooms is the fact that it is based on an understandable content that transcends cultural specificity, making emoji useful as transfer-learning devices that do not impede understanding of content because of cultural differences – in effect, they are effective learning artifacts that can be used as a basis for positive transfer. When students belong to the same speech community, as was typically the case in the past, the instruction and didactic devices required to interact strategically with them were based on a common core of cultural notions and references. But when students belong to different speech communities and cultures, as well as to different levels of development, the teaching process becomes a much more complex one. As Klyukanov (2005: 21) has aptly observed, in such settings, people tend to "define their collective identities by drawing boundary lines between themselves, looking for a mutually acceptable boundary fit." Klyukanov (2005: 60) goes on to note that cultural identity shapes the course of any interaction, since it is channeled through the language used:

> When people communicate with one another, they try to reach their goals by using various language means. Every act of communication is a performance whereby people face each other (either literally or in a mediated fashion, such as via telephone or the Internet) and, as if on stage, present themselves – their very identities – dramatically to each other.

The key pedagogical finding of the Petcoff study is that emoji literacy constitutes an out-of-school second literacy, as Ede and Lunsford (2009) call it, shaping user identities that can be incorporated into the classroom to teach literacy via the activation of transfer mechanisms. Given that some emoji have negative connotations that would likely upset the congeniality that is required for effective teaching and learning, the teacher should be aware of the fact that all sign systems are in a constant state of flux. Emoji such as the thumbs-up one or even the heart one, for example, may be inappropriate in certain contexts. Needless to say, this can happen in any classroom, where the out-of-class environment shapes meaning systems in ways to which the in-class world should respond. Actually, the Petcoff project showed that the classroom itself would inform the instructor as to what is appropriate or not, since it came up consistently. One should also be aware that overusing emoji may diminish their pedagogical efficacy (Berard 2018). All that said, the Petcoff study showed that emoji-based training presents opportunities for empowerment of disadvantaged or challenged students as they attempt to gain academic literacy.

Bimodality

Psychologically, the transfer from emoji literacy (visual understanding) to academic literacy (verbal understanding) can be viewed as a modal flow process, whereby it activates a flow of learning from visuality to verbality, corresponding to a coordination of the functions of the right hemisphere, where visuality is processed, with those of the left hemisphere, where most of the language functions are located.

Bimodality theory was originally conceived as a pedagogical construct aiming to apply neuroscientific theories and research to foreign language teaching (Danesi 1986, 2003). It was based on neuroscientific evidence that visual input involves the experiential right-hemisphere functions, which are called R-Mode, while verbal input activates the analytical capacities of the left hemisphere, designated L-Mode. In processing a hybrid text, therefore, the two modes are (presumably) activated in a continuous fashion, rather than in discrete stages. The bimodal processing of emoji has, actually, been documented by neuroscience. For example, Churches et al. (2014), used electrodes attached to the scalps of twenty subjects, asking them to look at actual faces and emoji, such as 🙂 for a smile and 🙁 for a frown. They also asked the participants to look at the same signs in inverted form: an upside-down face, for instance, or an emoji oriented the wrong way. The researchers found that when in their correct orientation, emoji are processed in the same occipitotemporal sites as face recognition within the temporal lobe located in both cerebral hemispheres, and the processing involves projecting sensory input into derived meanings for the appropriate retention of visual memory, language comprehension, and emotion association. In effect, emoji activate R-Mode and L-Mode functions in tandem. In another relevant study, Chatzichristos et al. (2020) collected fMRI data that indicated that hybrid structures (word + emoji) activated a number of areas spread throughout the brain, including the supplementary motor area, inferior prefrontal cortex, which is involved in the orchestration of thoughts, language, and planning, controlling various aspects of language and cognition, Broca's area (where most of the speech functions originate), the amygdala, and the right temporal pole. Again, this type of research supports the bimodality hypothesis put forth here – namely, that emoji activate R-Mode and L-Mode functions in a holistic fashion.

So, during the initial stages of learning to control literacy structures and meanings, bimodality theory suggests that students need to assimilate novel input through creative R-Mode activities, more so than other kinds of activities, which was corroborated by the Petcoff study. After this stage, students will benefit from formal literacy training, as part of L-Mode processing to reinforce what they have learned, including a creative use of hybrid writing that requires their background knowledge applied to novel input – another bimodal feature confirmed by the Petcoff study. Overall, the latter showed that: (1) experiential-creative forms of learning and teaching, with emoji, are R-Mode teaching strategies; (2) L-Mode literacy teaching should be deployed in tandem; and (3) the creative utilization of hybrid and traditional literacy allows students to move back and forth between different modes (R-Mode or L-Mode) fluidly.

Bimodality-based pedagogy makes one initial demand on teachers – it requires them to identify a specific learning task as being novel or not, and thus to apply bimodal techniques as needed. Generally speaking, something is novel when it involves structures or concepts that are either different or absent from the point at which the students find themselves. Suffice it to say that any task or input can be considered to be novel if the students demonstrate an inability to understand it or use it functionally. If that is so, instructional techniques that focus on rational analysis will be of little value, since the students have no preexisting L-Mode schemas for accommodating the new information directly. In order to make something accessible to the L-Mode, pedagogical experience dictates that the learner should be allowed to explore the new structures and concepts through R-Mode techniques. If, for example, the verbal tense system is an early objective of literacy training, then an R-Mode device that can help students grasp the relation can be the use of emoji in an episodic and recursive fashion, which allows for the student to perceive an isomorphism between verb use and the emoji annotation of time. While the students may not possess the formal knowledge of tense, they will nevertheless be able to grasp the meaning intuitively through the R-Mode and then map it against the formal L-Mode verbal structures accordingly. This can be bolstered by teacher input, as the students progress toward a solution conceptually, as was done in the Petcoff study. Once the initial R-Mode acquisition stage has been allowed to "run its course," the teacher can then "shift modes" and put the students in a frame of mind that allows them to reflect on the new structural patterns *in themselves* – involving the control of grammar.

Bimodality theory is also in line with the Vygotskian notion of zones of proximal development (mentioned earlier). To allow the R-Mode of the students to process the novel input expansively, such as the McWhorter video, they were asked to provide variations to the text creating their own interpretations via the basic paragraph and hybrid writing formats, no matter how many grammatical errors they might commit in the process. These can always be adjusted in a briefing session in class after the bimodal process has occurred. This secondary stage in the flow cannot be circumvented. L-Mode knowledge will not emerge on its own in a de facto manner. Obviously, some types of learners will need fewer formal explanations and reinforcement practice than others. Moreover, the type of instruction to be used will vary according to both learner cognitive style and type of input. The way to determine what modal technique is appropriate is for the teacher to simply to try one out, as did Petcoff. Clearly, if some activity does not seem to work, then another one (or a different one within the same general pedagogical approach) must be considered. Similarly, the degree of utilization of the students' background knowledge will depend on the level of competence reached by them – the more they are familiar with the new concept, the more the new material can be explained without bimodal strategies. Commentaries on any pattern or feature related to, or derived from, the new content should be elaborated when required.

What the Petcoff study also showed was that, at various points in the learning process, individual students may manifest some persistent difficulty in utilizing a concept or verbal structure (grammatical or lexical). At other points, they may show difficulty in using a certain concept in discourse. At such points, it is obvious that they will need to focus on the concept itself. In effect, there will be points in the learning flow when students may need to stop and focus on certain aspects of the material introduced.

It should be noted that bimodality theory is not new; rather, it encapsulates the classic work done on intuitive, inductive, and other forms of "open" learning, adapting it neuroscientifically. R-Mode learning corresponds by and large to implicit learning, defined as the learning of complex information in an incidental manner, without awareness of what has been learned (Frensch and Rünger 2003). Implicit learning requires a minimal amount of attention, depending on attentional and working memory mechanisms – the R-Mode activates these mechanisms via the emoji input. L-Mode learning corresponds largely to explicit learning, or the conscious, intentional grasp of factual information and concepts (Tulving 1972).

Already in the 1940s, neuropsychologist Alexander Luria (1947) had suggested that there existed an inherent bimodal connectivity in functional task distribution that spanned the entire brain. Adopting Roman Jakobson's (1942) idea that the selection of linguistic units and their combination were neurologically complementary processes, Luria showed that the latter were impaired by lesions in the anterior areas of the language centers, whereas the former were disrupted when damage occurred to the posterior areas of the same centers. Subsequent neuroscientific studies have confirmed Luria's findings, including studies utilizing computer models, which are designed to show how brain networks interconnect with each other in the processing of information. As Obler and Gjerlow (1999: 11) have put it, "there are no language centers per se but rather 'network nodes' that are stimulated; eventually one of these is stimulated enough that it passes a certain threshold and that node is 'realized,' perhaps as a spoken word."

One of the more relevant findings from neuroscience that is of direct relevance to the present discussion is that the right hemisphere is, in fact, a crucial "point-of-departure" for processing novel stimuli: that is, for handling input for which there are no preexistent cognitive codes or programs available. Already in the early 1980s, Goldberg and Costa (1981) suggested that the main reason why this is so is because of the anatomical structure of the right hemisphere. Its greater connectivity with other centers in the complex neuronal pathways of the brain makes it a better "distributor" of new information. The left hemisphere, on the other hand, has a more sequentially organized neuronal-synaptic structure and, thus, finds it more difficult to assimilate information for which no previous categories exist. No contradictory evidence has come forth since Goldberg and Costa's study. Actually, subsequent work has confirmed that the neuronal structures involved in bimodal processing are spread widely throughout the brain, primarily by neurotransmitters; and it now appears certain that different types of semiotic tasks activate different areas of the brain in many sequences and patterns. It has also become apparent that these are regulated, additionally, by the emotional areas of the brain. The limbic system – which includes portions of the temporal lobes, parts of the hypothalamus and thalamus, and other structures – has been found to play a larger role than previously thought in the processing of certain kinds of speech (Damasio 1994). Bimodality is, clearly, also consistent with Csíkszentmihályi's (1990) concept of learning flow, which claims that learners who are immersed in the learning process via creative activities tend to become highly motivated to explore their subject. As the Petcoff project showed, emoji-based activities can be seen as activating the flow naturally. A key study by Christofalos et al. (2020) confirmed that emoji can assume different relations with the sentence context in which they occur according to their bimodal valence. Using an online ratings task and a recognition memory task to determine if differences in emoji function within a sentence affect judgments of emoji-text coherence and subsequent recognition accuracy, the researchers found that emoji allow readers to extract relevant information (an R-Mode function) and then "integrate it with surrounding passage content" (an L-Mode function).

Overall, neuroscience has established that the brain's two hemispheres differ not so much as to the type of stimuli they are designed anatomically to process, as to the manner in which they process information. This is why it is improper, if not misleading, to use terms such as "right brain learning" or "left brain learning." These oversimplify the brain's mechanisms involved in processing input. Terms such as L-Mode and R-Mode, on the other hand (as initially proposed by Edwards 1979), are preferable because they refer only to types of processes associated with one or the other hemisphere, but not exclusively so. Contemporary brain-scanning research has shown that while each hemisphere is specialized to handle a specific type of function, it does so in tandem with complementary or parallel processing patterns taking place in the other hemisphere and in other parts of the brain. While this might appear to be an oversimplification of how the brain works, it can be argued that it nonetheless is highly useful as a framework for grasping how developmental students were able to shift from intuitive R-Mode forms of understanding to more formal L-Mode forms in the case of academic literacy. Overall, emoji spontaneously initiate a modal flow, allowing students to focus on content and (subsequently) on its relation to form (verbal and visual). The effectiveness of emoji can be discerned in the fact that: (1) they are R-Mode signs that introduce content through a creative-visual format that engages students in a classroom dialectic; (2) they allow for L-Mode reflection on the connection between their visual form and the content on which they are based; and (3) they allow for a back and forth between these two modal systems. An analogy to music teaching can perhaps be made here to illustrate the practical implications of bimodality theory. Learning how to play a new piece on the piano, say, entails the ability to mold the component mechanical skills needed to play the notes, phrases, and so on of the piece successfully into the global skill of "playing the music." But, in order to give the learner's L-Mode a better opportunity to organize the component skills into automatic psychomotor routines, the teacher normally starts out by playing the piece for the student, making appropriate aesthetic comments here and there, relating these to the techniques needed to successfully execute the new piece. In this way, the student's R-Mode has an opportunity to decipher the new musical input in a global aesthetic way. The component mechanical skills can then be understood separately and practiced apart from their role in the music. Needless to say, an advanced piano student who is already in firm control of the required L-Mode skills through previous training will not have to spend as much time on this orientation phase as would a beginner. When students have mastered the L-Mode aspects of the piece, then they will be in a position to integrate them with the R-Mode ones as they perform the piece. A consummate performance of the piece is, from a neurological perspective, a bimodal feat, requiring the integrated contribution of both the R-Mode and the L-Mode to the performative task at hand.

Students store tasks that have been acquired creatively in long-term memory, and when new information is presented to them, they search instinctively for associations that link the new information with what they have learned in memory. The associative system in the brain thus reinforces the new information and assigns meaning to it. Of special relevance is the role of emoji in activating associative processes, allowing them to seek meaning in the input between what would otherwise be perceived as mere information. As is widely known, this is called *priming*, whereby exposure to one domain of knowledge influences a response to subsequent information, without conscious guidance (Bargh and Chartrand 2000; McDonough and Trofimovich 2008).

Epilogue

The overall conclusion that can be reached in using emoji for some educational task, such as imparting literacy to developmental learners, is that they activate a bimodal process of learning, without interrupting the background knowledge that students bring to class. When imparting academic literacy, as the Petcoff study showed, at the very least it is much easier to center the teaching process on what the students already know. This not only renders the learning process relevant to student experiences but is also psychologically effective for reasons such as those discussed in this chapter. The use of emoji literacy as the transfer mechanism toward traditional literacy is a practical answer to the very gnarled problem of how to impart literacy to developmental students, given the kind of communicative environment in which we are all immersed. The question of whether emoji literacy can be used in other areas of education will be broached in Chapter 6. It should also be noted that the notion of bimodality is consistent with the notion of conceptual blending in neuroscience (Fauconnier and Turner 2002; Oakley and Pascual 2017), which proposes that different areas of the brain are mapped against each other in producing novel ideas.

As the Petcoff study showed, the use of the emoji code in a formal pedagogical way allows the teacher to overcome many of the past barriers when it came to developmental students, because it speaks to them in their own way, helping engage them by breaking down complicated subject matter that may seem worlds away to them. As bimodal theory suggests, moreover, they create an environment that activates an inbuilt "sensorium," as McLuhan (1962) claimed – namely, an amalgam of sensation, perception, and interpretation of information about the world around us. McLuhan claimed that our senses are activated differentially by the diverse media. In the case of a new medium, such as emoji, the sensorium is reconstituted, retrieving some of the qualities of orality (as discussed). In early cultures, people lived in an acoustical–tactile sensorium through which they understood the world. With the advent of alphabets and the literate mind, the sensorium in which people lived and thought became highly visual and abstract. The print age favored this type of cognition, putting value on reading versus listening. In the modern-day world, there is a retrieval of many of the sensory patterns of the oral world, blending verbality and visuality in a new way. The introduction of emoji into pedagogy is a way to create a sensorium that is in sync with the way we actually communicate in the global village, to use another of McLuhan's well-known terms.

Given the presentational, recursive, discursive, and visual literacy properties of emoji, their educational operationality transverses and transcends disciplines, modalities, and languages. While instructors of developmental education, first-year writing, postsecondary writing, and rhetoric are the primary audience for the Petcoff study, there is little doubt that the use of emoji in classrooms will have relevance in multiple pedagogical areas. Some of these are discussed subsequently.

3 Emoji in Healthcare Communications and Education

Prologue

As studies on the use of emoji in education have made evident (discussed in Chapter 6), emoji are not just ancillary pedagogical devices that can spruce up a classroom in a comic book way but rather tap into a bimodal flow of thinking that enhances the learning process (Freedman 2014; Mills, Stone and Unsworth 2020). As the Petcoff study showed (Chapter 2), a primary reason why emoji activate this process optimally is that they are already a part of the communicative competence of not only literacy-challenged students but also other students, given that they are accustomed to the routine, systematic use of emoji in everyday digital communications. This might explain why emoji have entered classrooms across the disciplinary spectrum, as teachers intuitively sense their usefulness as part of an ever-expanding multimedia literacy that students use creatively to make themselves understood in new, sophisticated ways. Shannon Correia (2021) sums up the situation aptly: "Emojis have become second nature when texting. From rising out of a need to express emotion over text messages, these icons have changed the way we communicate digitally."

One area that is of interest in emoji use is medicine and healthcare, given that the way patients and practitioners communicate with each other is often crucial in influencing the success of a therapeutic or medical strategy. As seen in Chapter 2, communications among lay persons are clearer when they are communicated with emoji, in contrast to attempts to fit thoughts into linguistic communication structures specific to other cultures (much like medical lingo that is not easily understood by the general public). Research has shown, in fact, that effective physician–patient communication will positively influence health outcomes by increasing patient understanding of health problems and treatments available, contributing to a better attitude toward adherence to treatment plans, and providing support and reassurance via the visual nature of emoji themselves. In 1992, Ezekiel and Linda Emanuel proposed four models for the physician–patient relationship: the paternalistic, interpretive, deliberative, and informative models, which differ according to the perception of the goal of physician–patient interactions, the physician's responsibilities, the role of patient values, and the concept of patient autonomy. Put forth in the era before the advent of emoji communication, the study suggested that the interpretive model was the most effective, given that it was based on a shared set of meanings delivered through commonly used forms. It is in the framework of this model that emoji usage in written patient–clinician communications would be located.

Healthcare is a relationship between clinician, patient, and system, focused on a patient's condition. Patient safety depends on this relationship. Trust, confidence, decision-making, error prevention and identification, and continuity of care in healthcare rely centrally on effective communication, with the patient the actual center to the conversations. Despite advances in patient charting systems, seeing a patient in person is crucial to providing appropriate care. Aside from physical examinations, in-person interactions allow for enhanced assessment, which is reinforced through the insights provided via nonverbal aspects of an interaction, as well as a better assessment of the patient's needs. In-person interactions build trust and rapport and foster opportunities to address patient concerns. Patient charts and in-person interactions provide, in tandem, a fuller picture of the patient. However, there are gaps in the picture that constantly emerge. Text messaging using emoji traverses electronic records and in-person interactions, acting as a conduit toward the development of a fuller picture of the patient's condition.

With the technological advances of mobile devices and the need for healthcare groups to communicate with a growing number of patients, patient–provider interactions have shifted to text messaging as a primary mode of communication. This eliminates follow-up visits and allows timely communication. It also serves as a reference system available for review that can reduce miscommunication, elevating its importance as a form of patient records. As technology continues to evolve and as the burden on healthcare systems increases, digital modes of communication are likely to play an increasingly integral role in patient access, patient-centered care, and engagement.

Studies have demonstrated that the approach taken by physicians to communicate information is as critical as the actual information itself, since it has been shown to influence emotional health, symptom resolution, pain control, blood pressure levels, and the like (Stewart 1995; Lee et al. 2002; Ha and Longnecker 2010). When miscommunication occurs, it can have negative consequences, reducing levels of patient hopefulness. This chapter will examine the use of emoji as an effective code for making physician–patient communication effective, given that it projects the emotivity structures of discourse into a dialectic that is inclusive of both addressers (practitioners) and addressees (patients and students). Moreover, they attenuate the stigma of not understanding professional jargon, encouraging participation on both sides. The chapter will also broach the use of emoji in training medical and public health practitioners, not only because it is a corollary to the generic educational goal of this book but also because emoji can provide more specifically a means to optimize student–teacher and student–student interactions. The underlying premise here is that fluency in emoji use is becoming essential to healthcare. It is the same premise that undergirded the Petcoff study (Chapter 2) – namely, emoji literacy is now an unconscious part of students' natural communicative habits and can thus be harnessed to enhance the learning process at various levels, given the bimodal nature of hybrid communications.

The topic of this chapter thus falls, overall, under the rubric of semioliteracy applied to the healthcare field – encompassing the use of multimedia artifacts in this area and highlighting the hybrid emoji code, in both health professions interactions and in the training of clinicians. Interestingly, the connection between semiotics, the study of signs, and medicine goes back to antiquity and was elaborated concretely by John Locke, who was both a physician and philosopher, in his *Essay Concerning Humane Understanding* (Locke 1690), in which he revived the Hippocratic term *semeiotics* (referring to the study of symptoms originally), defining it as a method of inquiry based on what has been called here semioliteracy – the ability to use all kinds of signs (verbal and nonverbal) in the construction of messages of different types. It is not clear where Locke got the idea to use the original Hippocratic term, although he was a medical doctor – the term was used two decades earlier in 1670 by the English physician Henry Stubbe to designate the interpretation of signs within and outside of medicine (Deely 2001). Locke's proposal, however, did not catch on broadly. As is well known, the birth of a veritable science of signs had to await the Swiss philologist Ferdinand de Saussure (1916), who called it semiology instead and, in America, the logician Charles S. Peirce (1931–1958), who provided a technical lexicon for discussing the different kinds of signs used in different media.

Emoji and Well-Being

A premise that can be put forth is that emoji in physician–patient interactions and in actual clinical settings have the self-contained ability to promote well-being in themselves (Danesi 2022). The argument is that this is a likely effect of the general positive emotivity function of emoji. To reiterate, it was Roman Jakobson (1960) who saw emotivity as one of the fundamental discourse-semiotic functions of communicative interactions, conveying emotional states, sentiments, points of view, opinions, and feelings, either explicitly in discourse choices or implicitly in the subtext of a discourse. As discussed, emotivity is intrinsic to understanding the nature of facial emoji, which are intended, at one level, to represent facial expressions with iconically simplified signifiers, such as a slanted line to represent the lips curved up or down to stand for happiness or sadness respectively, but at another level to suggest state of mind or to project a subjective evaluation of the content of a message. Despite variability in terms of contextual, situational, cultural, and various other interpretations of facial emoji, the range of meaning is nonetheless constrained by their everyday similar functions in global communications, where a common ground of semiotic understanding has crystallized through the intercultural usage of the emoji – a semiotic compromise necessitated by the need to make global communications as commonly comprehensible as possible. The smiley emoji is, thus, typically perceived to convey some degree of happiness within the conceptual context of a digital message and the tears emoji to communicate the feeling of sadness, with variation that has been widely documented. Such emoji reduce the physical facial expressions engendered by certain emotions to their bare outlines, with apposite signifiers. By removing other features of the face that would intervene in the interpretive process, such emoji constitute a kind of "agreed-upon" meaning pattern that, however, can be used for ironic or some other discursive intent, so that it can have sarcastic or negative meaning, depending on message content and context of use.

So, there seems to have emerged a kind of consensus on what facial emoji mean that users from diverse background grasp unconsciously, or at least to which they agree for the sake of communicative fluidity. Obviously, those who feel offended by some emoji will avoid using it but if it is sent to them likely now understand the positive intent of the sender, thus ignoring the negativity. What originally started out as a small, pixelated set of pictograms has now become an intrinsic part of a modern global culture impacting day-to-day communication. As Gibson and colleagues (2018) found, predictably, one can never assume that an emoji has an inherent, universal meaning. This is, of course, true of any sign form in any language. However, the difference is that the range of variability is more constrained in emoji usage, especially given their constant usage in all kinds of communications. In the end, the study concluded that the emoji code is a global component of written language with predictable limits. So, a smiley emoji can be used for emphasizing joy in a given text message, while it may have an ironic meaning in another message. But overall, there is an understanding that the meaning of a smiley has a limited emotive range. So, when a text message has smiley faces inserted throughout, it is almost impossible to interpret it as conveying anything but a positive emotivity, unless it is intended to be ironic or sarcastic – which can be gleaned by reading the intent of the entire message. The conveyance of sentiment is unconscious. And the argument can be made that, because of this, facial emoji can detect states or levels of well-being in patients.

Corroborative studies include the following:

- A study by Lee et al. (2008) used emoji as less time-consuming tools for detecting depression after stroke. They found that the sad emoji showed a high agreement rate with the Diagnostic and Statistical Manual for Major Depression, indicating that, along with other sentiment emoji, the smiley could be used for screening depression among patients.
- A study by O'Reilly-Shah et al. (2018) found that the use of emoji as substitutes for words to augment technical medical communications facilitated such communication considerably. However, there were some disadvantages connected with the lack of standardization of emoji form and style on different platforms, variability of cultural meaning, and conveyance of unintended meanings.
- Willoughby and Liu (2018) found that using emoji in health-related messages is more effective in conveying the objectives and content of the messages than print text. Attention was enhanced when emoji were added to weaker and less interesting verbal health texts.
- A 2018 paper published in the *Journal of Oncology* (Thomson et al. 2018) found that emoji were a comprehensible, reliable measurement of cancer patient-reported outcomes, especially for subjects with low health literacy. Of the seventy-five patients who took part in the study, 92 percent reported they would use emoji scales again and 89 percent would recommend their use to others.
- A 2019 study (Marengo et al. 2019) found that emoji accurately identified symptoms of depression in over 400 young adults.
- A 2020 study of English and Spanish-speaking people (Stonbraker et al. 2020), most of them with low health literacy, found that a bar graph combined with emoji was the preferred format of the subjects, given that it was the easiest for them to understand.
- In another 2020 study (Lotfinejad et al. 2020), it was found that emoji encourage the use of hand hygiene in stemming the spread of antimicrobial resistance.

In a way, the research has come forth to empirically support Susanne Langer's (1948) view that there is an inherent connection between human feeling and visual representation, leading her to construct a theory of feeling as a psycho-biological process that humans express through various forms of representation. She also saw human dialogue as designed to connect our emotional reactions to words (and other symbols) in an unconscious fashion, shaping how we react to interlocutors. This is similar to Mikhail Bakhtin's (1981) view that dialogue is implanted (unconsciously) in emotivity, whereby interlocutors create and present their subjective realities (explicitly or implicitly), which in turn shapes Self–Other relations. Dialogical interactions are not constrained to convey information objectively; rather, many arise from a need to communicate affective experiences among interlocutors, rather than just to relay specific information, ideas, point of view, and so on. It is thus emotive in its psychological foundations. Emoji tap into this form of inherent emotivity in an effective way, implicating feeling structures, rather than rational-informational ones. The branch of semiotics into which they can be located, more concretely, is *significs*, or the study of signs and sign systems as based on sensations, feelings, impressions, and other emotive states. The term is traced to Lady Victoria Welby (1897), who, as Susan Petrilli (2009) has shown in great detail, understood that many signs spring from emotional-sensory reactions to the world rather than just information-gathering and classificatory needs. Without going into details here, suffice it to say that significs allows us to connect sense, meaning, and significance in emoji usage. The former is essentially the expressive-sensory element in all experience; even in "senseless" speech its "grains" are latent, as Welby noted. Meaning is a kind of refinement of sense: that is, it is purposive sense. Finally, significance is, essentially, a blending of sense and meaning, but transcending the blend itself in range and implication.

Consider the typical smiley within this framework. As such, it evokes an affective form of sense-making, representing a basic emotion in outline form, namely, happiness or joy (to some degree); but its significance transcends this simple communicative aspect, since it delves into how it might function in human life as a metaphor of human experiential events and needs (Figure 3.1).

As Petrilli (2009) has shown, these three dimensions are not sequential but rather holistically intertwined, involving an array of semiotic processes, including implication, connotation, figuration, and so on. An informal study (Danesi 2022) revealed how students assess the smiley in signific terms, ranging in responses from happiness to ironic stance, confirming its use as an emotive signifier. The subjects also maintained that the smiley was an indication of well-being. We speak of going through trials and tribulations; we never speak of going through well-being. As Welby pointed out, the former is an external state that can be described in concrete ways, as if it were a metaphorical object existing in time and space; the latter is instead an internal state

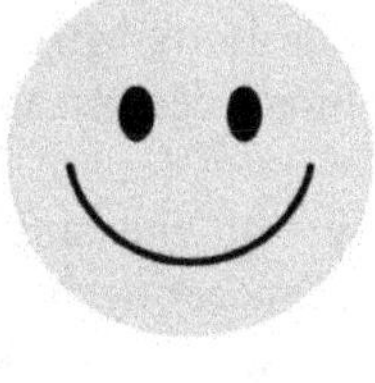

Figure 3.1 Typical smiley (MS Office Shape)

that is permanent in the emotional makeup of the subject. It is much harder to express in verbal language. It is in this sense that emoji are effective in expressing internal states – a premise for which there is ample empirical support. For example, Lu et al. (2022) found that smileys help better monitor the well-being of remote workers. Using machine learning to track how the emoji were being used in online conversations, the researchers found that people who regularly used facial emoji to convey their emotions at work would have better emotional health, regardless of whether the emoji they used were positive or negative. This was then converted into higher engagement and less likelihood that the worker would leave the project or the platform.

The history of the smiley can actually be traced to antiquity. Archaeologists have discovered a Hittite pot, from approximately 1700 BCE, in Karkemish, Turkey, which had a large smiling face engraved on it, resembling in outline form the modern-day emoji figure (Marchetti 2015). Around 500 BCE, the Greeks created two masks representing smiling and frowning faces, representing the theatrical genres of comedy and tragedy respectively. While more elaborate in style, they are clearly suggestive of the contemporary emoji faces. Similar masks are found throughout the ancient world, having come down to us in the form of ritualistic carnival masks with different design features. Commercial uses of a smiling face figure imprinted on stickers started emerging in the 1920s in the United States. The first true predecessor of the yellow smiley emoji is traced to 1962, when radio station WMCA in New York City released a sweatshirt with a yellow smiley figure design as part of a marketing campaign. A number of T-shirt designers subsequently created yellow happy faces over the next few decades. During the counterculture peace movement of the 1960s, the smiley came to be used as a symbol of peace – a symbolism adopted as well by subsequent youth cultures. By 1972, Frenchman Franklin Loufrani had legally trademarked the yellow happy face, calling it "Smiley" for the first time. Loufrani argued that the design was so simple that no one person could lay claim to having created it, pointing to early cave paintings found in France that, he maintained, exhibited the first depictions of a similar face. Nonetheless, he trademarked it. The smiley made its appearance on the Internet for the first time in September of 1982, when computer scientist Scott Fahlman at Carnegie Mellon University suggested that the emoticon :-) be read sideways to mean that a statement was a joke. By 1993, the smiley face was finally included by Unicode in its Miscellaneous Symbols version 1.1. Since then, it has become *the* most recognizable emoji across the globe.

The point of the foregoing brief historical foray into the smiley is to emphasize that a sign does not emerge in a void, but rather derives its current form and cumulative meanings from previous phases. Polish-American scholar Alfred Korzybski (1921) designated this aspect of meaning-making a "time-binding" characteristic, defined as the capacity of an individual or a generation to begin where the former left off. The presence of the smiley since antiquity is connected to some form of happiness (including comedy and laughter), which suggests that it has always been associated with well-being in a time-binding (across generations) way. Wiseman and Gould (2018), for instance, found that the use of emoji in digital communications conveyed a wealth of emotions that otherwise would take many words to express. They were also repurposed for something other than their intended use between close partners, family members, and friends. So, certain emoji might get chosen because they are meaningful to the specific interlocutors – that is, they are used to convey intimate and personal sentiments that, for various reasons, cannot be expressed easily (or economically) in words, thus becoming part of an unconscious communicative episodic grammar (discussed further in Chapter 7). Needless to say, the problem of ascribing a common set of emotive meanings to emoji is fraught with difficulty, given the presence of variation and the subjective uses that emoji use might entail. For example, the grinning face emoji 😁 constitutes an unsure and precarious reaction to some content. This emanates typically from an episodic mode of understanding, guided by the location of the emoji in relation to other emoji, which provides an interpretative frame for decoding the meaning of the sign.

The late writer and social critic Susan Sontag cogently argued in her compelling 1978 book, *Illness as Metaphor*, that the ways in which we speak about a disease predisposes us to perceive it in specific ways, since the words created and utilized historically to describe it might have moral judgments built into them of which we are not consciously aware. The words are thus potential psychosomatic triggers that affect not only how we think about an illness but also how we might react to it physically and even medically. Choosing *le mot juste*, as Hippocrates and Locke suggested, is an essential part of a diagnostic semiotic approach to physical and mental disease; and it is in this sense that emoji might have the capacity to facilitate therapy, since they constitute not *le mot juste*, but *l'image juste.* Skiba (2016) was one of the first to look at the health implications of using emoji, reviewing the relevant psycho-therapeutic literature that suggested that graphic or infographic symbolism facilitated health literacy and engaged patients with their own health perceptions. Given the growing use of mental health apps, Skiba claimed that practitioners could help eliminate the health literacy divide, since emoji are perceived as relatively free from the judgmental aspects of some words in this domain. She makes the following relevant observation (Skiba 2016: 57): "Imagine if nursing were to develop a set of emoji that could be used in the care of patients and allow patients to better understand and communicate their challenges with managing their health. There are lots of emoji for emotions, but there are relatively few, if any, that are health related." Van Dam et al.

(2019) looked at how the use of emoji can help young people with mental health problems cope with them better. Using the technique of ecological momentary assessment, based on extracting data from smartphones, they were able to better predict risks of behavioral and health problems for (self-monitoring) interventions. The researchers collected data from thirty-two participants (aged 16–24) with mental health issues, over a three-month period, and interviewed a subsample of ten adolescents who received psychological therapy. The results indicated that the emoji in the apps could identify positive and negative feelings, as well as individual symptom patterns, rather accurately. However, there was a caveat. While adolescents receiving mental healthcare were very positive about applications of the emoji-based indicators, there was always the possible drawback of inaccurate representation and incorrect predictions of emotional states, given the fact that emoji meanings are continually changing on the Internet.

Another relevant study of emoji use to promote well-being in children is the one by Jennifer Fane (2017), which involved the use of emoji as a child-centered method for eliciting young children's perspectives of their own well-being. The findings of the study suggested that many children are able to articulate their own understanding and experiences of well-being using emoji, rather than verbal language. This study provides a rationale for the use of child-centered tools to facilitate children's exploration and communication of their own understanding and experiences of well-being. A study by Siegel et al. (2015) on 297 elementary school children produced similar results, finding that the placement of green smiley faces on milk and vegetable products increased the children's desire to consume them.

In the Hippocratic corpus, the notion of *symptom* is treated with great sophistication and cultural sensitivity. The physician must take into account the symptom's intensity and frequency, as well as the stage of the disease that it indicates. The physician must also take directly into account the social and psychological characteristics of the patient – age, habits, speaking style, and so on – in tandem with the strictly diagnostic aspects of an examination. The overarching principle in the Hippocratic corpus is that a symptom must be considered not in isolation but rather in combination with other factors, physical, subjective, and cultural. In this way, the meanings of symptoms can be determined by the physician's *gnóme* ("interpretation"), which consists of examining biological factors and using a comprehensible language (*gnōstá toĩsı dē mótēısın*) that allows the physician to converse with the patient so that the latter can provide useful information. Today, that language is more often than not the visual language of emoji. As Lin and You (2023) affirm: "By providing health information through visual communication, public health organizations can effectively guide and persuade people to adopt healthy behaviors, which is critical in the context of public health crises."

Practitioner–Patient Communications

The argument that emoji can enhance practitioner–patient interactions, especially in the case of young children, people with disabilities, and patients who speak other languages, is now a well-documented one, as discussed (and elaborated on further in Chapter 5). An effective dialogue between patient and practitioner is critical, as the Hippocratic corpus maintained, especially in the early stages of diagnosis. Consider facial acne, which is a dermatological condition linked largely to lifestyle factors (such as diet and stress). The most obvious symptom associated with this condition is the flareup of pimples (furuncles) on the face (and elsewhere). But these are not symptoms that define only acne – they can also be caused by hormonal changes or yeast infections, for example. So, the appearance of pimples may or may not be a sign of acne. Their linkage to the latter would come out through not only medical examination but also a dialogue with the sufferer, during which lifestyle factors, such as diet, would emerge as relevant or not. Given the stigma associated with pimples, especially in adolescence, the use of emoji to assuage the shame may be critical, as an anonymous perusal of tweets of acne sufferers has shown. Figure 3.2 is an example of what can be called an "acne-coping emoji."

As the foregoing discussion implies, part of the process of diagnosing a disease is a semiotic-dialogical one (Baer 1988). The use of emoji in this area is to allow patients to better understand and convey their symptoms, concerns, and other clinically relevant issues, as a study carried out by a group of physicians at the Massachusetts General Hospital, headed by Shuhan He, has suggested (Marzouk et al. 2022; Renne et al. 2022). Interestingly, the first medical emoji – the syringe and the pill – were introduced by Unicode in 2015. In 2017, Apple added emoji to represent people with disabilities, followed by emoji for the stethoscope, bones, teeth, and microbes in 2019. He and his group have added considerably to the list, including emoji for the liver, the kidneys, an MRI machine, and a white blood cell, among others. Semiotic problems have emerged in this communicative domain, as anticipated. In addition to how a patient may interpret or misinterpret, say, the emoji of a kidney, there is the problem of what a kidney emoji should look like. Would it include the

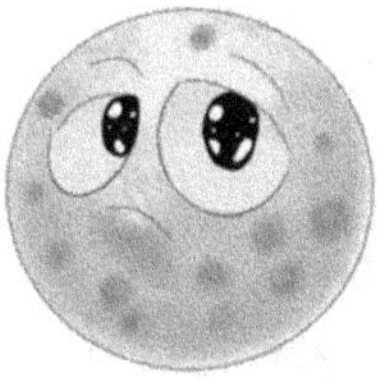

Figure 3.2 Acne emoji

blood vessels? Should it depict one kidney or the pair? Would the average layperson even know what a kidney looks like? All that can be said is that, as in any applications of emoji to specific situations, the relation between form and content will have to be taken into consideration, so as to assay which features will be relevant to both patient and practitioner. The interpretant (as mentioned) is always a powerful shaper of semiosis and needs always to be taken into account in all dialogical interactions.

As Kashish Sharma (2023) has aptly observed, after reviewing relevant studies on the use of emoji in physician–patient communications, emoji "allow the patients to communicate symptoms and other relevant information in a better way … This might also pull down the language barrier that might exist between a doctor and a patient." The following table demonstrates a hypothetical example of how a written exchange of messages between a psychotherapist and a patient might be written in both a traditional print-only way and in a hybrid way, with the practitioner being (artificially) the one using emoji exclusively in this example. (Note that this is a made-up interaction, not an actual conversation; it is used merely for illustration.)

	No emoji		With emoji
Therapist:	For how long have you had these nightmares?	Therapist:	⏳ have you had these 😴 😱?
Patient:	Since I was a child.	*Patient*:	Since I was a child.
Therapist:	Do you know why?	*Therapist*:	😟?
Patient:	No.	*Patient*:	No.
Therapist:	Let me ask you a few questions: Do you feel inadequate in some area of your life?	*Therapist*:	Let me ask you a few ❓: Do you feel 😩 in some area of your life?
Patient:	I am not sure.	*Patient:*	I am not sure.
Therapist:	In your marriage, job, or family, for instance?	*Therapist:*	In your 💍, 👨‍💼, or 👪, for instance?
Patient:	Occasionally in my job.	*Patient:*	Occasionally in my job.
Therapist:	Do you know what makes you nervous on the job?	*Therapist:*	Do you know what makes you 😰 😬 on the 👨‍💼?
Patient:	I fear that others see me as incompetent.	*Patient:*	I fear that others see me as incompetent.
Therapist:	Do you think you are?	*Therapist:*	Do you 🤔 you are ⁉
Patient:	I guess.	*Patient:*	I guess.
Therapist:	Everyone feels this way. There are ways around this.	*Therapist:*	Everyone feels this way 😔. There are ways around this.
Patient:	Oh, what should I do?	*Patient:*	Oh, what should I do?
Therapist:	Maybe you can talk to your colleagues about it. Ask them why they believe what they do.	*Therapist:*	Maybe you can 🗣 to your colleagues about it. Ask them why they believe what they do.

	No emoji		With emoji
Patient:	OK. What should I ask them?	*Patient:*	OK. What should I ask them?
Therapist:	Be straightforward and diplomatic; simply ask "What should I do to improve?"	*Therapist:*	Be straightforward and diplomatic; simply ask "What should I do to improve?"
Patient:	Yes, I see where you are going. Will this get rid of my nightmares?	*Patient:*	Yes, I see where you are going. Will this get rid of my nightmares?
Therapist:	There is a good chance that it will.	*Therapist:*	

Even to an untutored clinical eye, the emoji-based script can be seen (literally) to flesh out underlying issues in the patient's mind that are causing difficulties, as well as conveying an implicit sensitivity to these issues on the part of our hypothetical therapist. It is the visual humorous annotations of the emoji that make the dialogue fluid therapeutically, presumably making the patient cope better emotionally with the problems. The nightmare emoji lightens up the situation at the very start, without diminishing its diagnostic significance, imbuing the whole message distributively. The pensive face emoji reinforces the idea that the therapist's questions are nonthreatening, but still designed to unravel the underlying problems. The marriage, job, and family emoji depict these referents in concrete ways. The nervous face emoji is an iconic representation of a face configured in a microexpression that shows what the sense of nervousness produces on the face; and the feeling down emoji is a way to show that this emotion is real, not exceptional. The talking emoji visually annotates the action of talking in a non-conflictual way. Finally, the crossed fingers emoji simply imparts a sense of good will and hope. It is relevant to note that if one did not know that this was a specific kind of interaction, the emoji would be virtually uninterpretable in themselves. Only in dialogical formats do the emoji signs assume a decipherable meaning.

Needless to say, the social relation between practitioner and patient must be a well-established and familiar one; otherwise, the emoji-based dialogue would be seen as ludicrous and even insulting. Moreover, the choice of the specific emoji is constrained as to their comprehensibility in the social context in which they are used. These would make little sense beyond this context; so it is the therapist who will have to be knowledgeable of the cultural aspects of a diagnostic interaction, as Hippocrates certainly understood. Given these constraints and caveats, the primary goal of the dialogue is to make a patient concretely aware of relevant background factors in their particular symptomatology (such as having nightmares). The dialogue, albeit hypothetical, is not unlike the kind that is used by actual psychotherapists. The idea of therapeutic dialoguing using emoji is, clearly, to flesh out any hidden emotions, desires, intents, and so on in a nonjudgmental way. As Freud maintained, there seem to be "unconscious mental acts" that we do not comprehend, and these might, purportedly, be sources of distress. The unconscious, according to Freud (1901), shapes our conscious behaviors, which are vulnerable to various emotional and irrational impulses within us that Freud categorized under the notion of the Id. Speaking directly about these impulses might put up an emotional barrier between therapist and patient. The argument made here is that the barrier can be removed, or at least lowered, via emoji communication. Freud described the Id as follows (quoted in Hinsie and Campbell 1970: 372):

> We can come nearer to the Id with images, and call it chaos, a cauldron of seething excitement. We suppose that is somewhere in direct contact with somatic processes, and takes over from them instinctual needs and gives them mental expression. These instincts fill it with energy but it has no organization and no unified will, only an impulsion to obtain satisfaction for the instinctual needs, in accordance with the pleasure-principle.

If this "cauldron of seething excitement" dominates us, then we have an abundance of energy that we cannot use because of social rules and constraints (the Superego), which provoke a conscience-taking impulse that is based in social rules. This is the cause of the suppression of sentiments, which, arguably, can be alleviated via a form of communication that is visually evocative. The Id seeks gratification and has great energy, but cannot be expressed freely because it must submit to the demands of society – demands that might cause considerable mental anguish. The goal of an emoji-based therapeutic dialogue is to pinpoint the sources of the anguish in a way that evokes a sense of jocularity that allows patients to engage with their unconscious and come to grips with what it provokes in their lives. Empirical research has come forth to lend support to the argument made here. Nustrat and Huang (2021), for example, found that when therapists used emoji, patients would tend to perceive them as more empathetic, which positively influenced their overall counseling experience. Liu and Sun (2021) even found associations between personality traits and people's reasons and patterns for using emoji. They discovered specifically that emoji can help people with different personality traits achieve different objectives in their daily communication. In a study of Spanish speakers using emoji, Ferré et al. (2022) cataloged the effects of emoji in terms of their perceived emotivity. The researchers surveyed more than 1,100 students from the Spanish cities of Tarragona and Madrid to rate a random selection of 1,031 emoji. The findings indicated that there was a high level of agreement in the dataset with regard to the emotions and meanings communicated by emoji – confirming a premise of this chapter. As Harper (2022) notes in discussing the overall research: "This suggests that, in general, people interpret emojis in similar ways … [and this] aligns modern use with the historical use of smileys in previous iterations of communication platforms."

In *The Science of Medicine*, Hippocrates stated: "What escapes our vision we must grasp by mental sight, and the physician, being unable to see the nature of the disease nor to be told of it, must have recourse to reasoning from the symptoms with which he is presented," which means that the main goal of diagnosis is to "deduce of what disease they (the symptoms) are the result, what has happened in the past and to prognosticate the future course of the malady" (cited in Chadwick and Mann 1950: 87–89). Hippocrates' statement implies that the patient's history, as revealed through diagnostic interactions, is part of prognostication. So, the question becomes: How can patient history and background be elicited in such a way as to maximize the effectiveness and accuracy of prognostication? First and foremost, this means that a scientific study of the modalities of speech may be required to shed light on the situation; and, as claimed here, this would entail understanding the form of emoji literacy that a patient brings to a diagnostic situation. Needless to say, there was no science of language or of hybrid communication in antiquity. The ancients were, nonetheless, keenly aware of the power of language in shaping beliefs, views, and even physical well-being. Current research in linguistics and semiotics has accumulated a vast corpus of findings on how speech in all its modalities affects cognition, social interactions, and well-being.

Taking his cue from the Danish philologist Otto Jespersen (1922), Roman Jakobson (1960) provided one of the first useful classifications of speech acts in terms of the constituents and functions that speech acts entail. Given the research on the positive effects of emoji usage on physician–patient interactions, it is worthwhile revisiting Jakobson's overall model, mapping it against the emoji-based hypothetical dialogue discussed earlier, as an exercise in corroboration. Jakobson started by positing that there were six constituents that must be present for any speech act to become realizable in the first place:

- *Addresser*. This is the person or entity who initiates a communicative interaction. As we saw with the hypothetical dialogue earlier, the addresser in this case is the practitioner who initiates a form of dialogue intended to get to the nature of the relevant symptomatology; it could also be the patient who wishes to communicate the conditions and situations that brought about the symptoms. The emoji help establish a visual medium of understanding that corresponds to everyday usage.
- *Message*. This is the content that the addresser creates in order to convey something to someone else. The interaction is structured as a Q&A (question-and-answer) format, which allows the addresser to elicit the relevant information from the addressee. As we saw earlier, the elicitation is less inelastic and much more amicable than the normal type of dialogue when emoji are inserted.

- *Addressee.* This is the intended receiver of the message. The addressee can be the patient, who needs to understand in concrete and practical terms what the physician is saying, or it can be the physician, who needs to interpret the patient's descriptions and observations in terms of their clinical relevance. In either case, the emoji constitute a visual language that conveys meaning in terms of a mutually understandable code.
- *Context.* This is the situation (psychological, physical, social, etc.) that provides the cues for interpreting the message correctly. For example, the exhortation *Help me* takes on a different meaning depending on whether it is uttered by someone lying motionless on the ground or by someone in a classroom who is working on a difficult math problem. The context for the dialogue seen earlier is the situation in which a mental state is identified and understood. Recall the case of acne. If the patient lives in a world where diet is a likely factor causing the symptomatology, then acne can be considered as the most likely malady; if not, then some other explanatory path must be opened up. Using appropriate emoji can both alleviate the stigma associated with acne and suggest solutions in simple yet important ways.
- *Contact.* This is the actual interactional medium (face-to-face, phone, social media, etc.) by which the message is delivered between an addresser and an addressee. The mode of contact is typically face-to-face, but with new digital technologies it can also occur through some digital platform and, in the case of self-diagnosis, through the consultation of websites such as WebMD. By using emoji, the contact mode is enlarged verbally and visually, expanding understanding in a bimodal way.
- *Code.* This is the sign system (language, gesture, emoji, etc.) providing the signs (paradigmatic structure) and the combinatory rules (syntagmatic structure) for encoding and decoding messages. The features of the emoji code discussed previously and elaborated further in subsequent chapters, such as their episodic and distributional qualities, will enhance physician–patient empathy.

Jakobson then identified six functions that define the relations between messages and interlocutors:

- *Emotive.* As discussed several times, this is the intent of the addresser in delivering the speech act. Emotivity thus comprises the addresser's emotions, attitudes, social status, and intent, which reveal cumulatively the reason or reasons why the addresser entered into a speech act in the first place. The emotive function is a crucial one, as we have reiterated throughout. In the situation where a serious illness such as cancer may be involved, the physician must attempt to attenuate the sense of hopelessness that the diagnosis might engender in a patient. This can be achieved through the medium of emoji.

- *Conative*. This is the effect (physical, psychological, social, etc.) that the message has, or is intended to have, on its receiver. The conative effect of the message is clearly critical in getting the patient to understand and cope with the ailment. This includes the appropriate style and content on the part of the physician, which in the case of emoji usage blends the two in a unique way via annotation.
- *Referential*. This is any message constructed to convey information unambiguously; it is also the term Jakobson used to imply the semiotic awareness that a message is perceived as referring to something other than itself ("Main Street is two blocks north of here"). The referential aspect of the message will provide the patient with the kinds of information that will likely aid successful treatment, which was conveyed as seen earlier with emoji such as the diplomatic and talk ones.
- *Poetic*. This is any message constructed to deliver meanings effectively, like poetry ("I like it, I like it"). The poetic function in this case involves the appropriate choice of emoji that can convey something like a visual poem (episodically).
- *Phatic*. This is any message designed to establish, acknowledge, or reinforce social relations ("Hi, how's it going?"). The phatic aspects of a clinical interaction involve using conversational cues that allow the patient to grasp the message in a psychologically meaningful yet nonjudgmental way.
- *Metalingual* (or *metalinguistic*). This is any message that refers to the code used ("The word *noun* is a noun"). The metalinguistic function of emoji can be seen in the ways in which they translate medical notions visually, making them more understandable.

Jakobson's model suggests that verbal interaction goes well beyond simple information transfer. Semiotically, this means that in a dialogue, it is not the denotative meaning of the signs in combination that is the operative mode, but rather the connotative mode that guides the overall interpretation. So, the meaning of an interaction is motivated and shaped by the setting, the message intent, the participants, and the goals of each interlocutor. This model can certainly be mapped against any act of diagnostic interaction, as a means of understanding "what is going on." The metalinguistic function is more significant than is usually assumed. Jargon allows physicians to communicate with each other effectively and unambiguously at a professional, scientific level. But this same kind of technical knowledge cannot be assumed in the case of a typical diagnostic interaction between patient and physician (unless, of course, the patient is also a physician or knowledgeable of medicine). Essentially, this implies a translation from one register (technical) to another (colloquial). In such communications, emoji can be used in tandem with the jargon as Table 3.1 shows, which contains both Unicode-lexicon and non-Unicode healthcare emoji (created for this book), selected for their suggestiveness:

Table 3.1 *Emoji counterparts*

Medical term	Common term	Emoji counterpart	Annotation
hematoma	blood clot	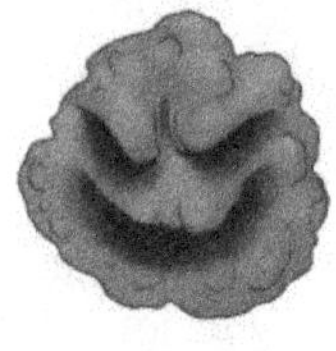	The personified angry heart emoji shows clumped red cells stopping circulation flow.
coronary thrombosis	heart attack	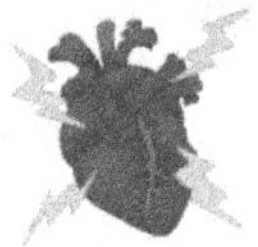	The emoji shows the heart undergoing thrombosis and thus needing immediate medical attention.
pruritis	itchiness	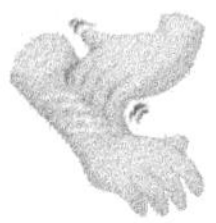	The scratching emoji plays on the sensation of physical itching and what it implies.
furuncle	boil, pimple	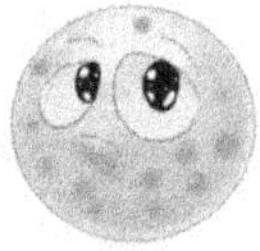	The worried, anxious look on the pimply-faced emoji is visually effective in bringing out the need to worry about the condition.
varicella	chickenpox	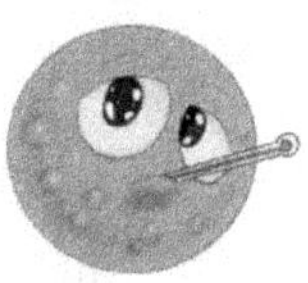	The emoji displays the symptoms of varicella and frames an emotive sad reaction, symbolized by green (a color associated with disease).
posology	dosage	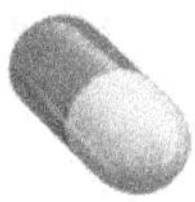	The pill emoji stands for dosage concretely.
strabismus	squinting	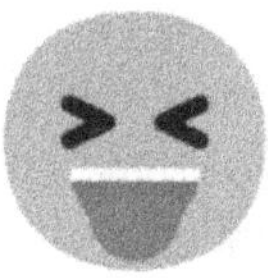	The squinting emoji adds a touch of humor to the experience of the condition, without downplaying the seriousness of the condition.
contusion	bruise	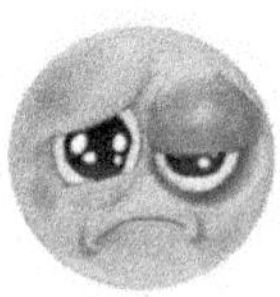	The bruised eye emoji connects bruising to a human cause (such as a punch).

We hardly realize the presence of the Jakobsonian mechanisms underlying communication. Traditionally, the study of how speech – spoken or written – unfolds via the deployment of these mechanisms has been relegated to either subsidiary status within linguistics or else considered to be more pertinently studied under some relevant branch. Research has shown, however, that speaking and writing are more than using language for various social purposes but are a means to relate to the world, to others, and to oneself. One of the general findings over the last half century is that sentences are not the basic units in language design. Rather, discourse texts are, as British-Australian linguist Michael Halliday (1985) abundantly documented. So, the parts of speech that make up sentences, such as pronouns, are more accurately described as "text-governed" structures, rather than items in a system of grammatical rules. Emoji are also text-governed in an episodic way, as discussed several times – that is, they provide a visual annotation to the event-episode structure of a message.

To sum up, as supported by a vast array of studies, the argument put forth here is that physician–patient writing communications can be rendered more effective through hybrid textuality (words and emoji). Emoji tend to render physician–patient dialogues effectively, positively influencing health outcomes by increasing patient satisfaction and even well-being. As healthcare evolves into a more personalized and patient-centered profession, the physician–patient relationship will become increasingly important. The personalized healthcare model encourages collaboration among physicians and patients in order to create shared health goals and the cultivation of agreed-upon health plans to address specific medical problems. By understanding the communicative factors that influence patient–physician relationships, healthcare providers will be able to address some of the barriers that might prevent patients from following prescribed medical treatments.

Image-Schematic Framing

As sociologist Erving Goffman (1978: 814) perceptively remarked, our utterances often make "a claim of sorts on the attention of everyone in the social situation." Deborah Tannen (1989) refers to a passage written by the famous anthropologist Gregory Bateson in which he remarks that in one of his writings he had attempted "to bring the reader into the room." Tannen (1989: 168) suggests that what Bateson is alluding to is a discourse strategy that constitutes "a way of achieving understanding through involvement." Goffman (1959, 1974) put forth the idea that how people talk about themselves indicates how they think about the world, introducing the method of *frame analysis* to study the relation between speech and personal understanding.

A similar type of analysis can also be used to understand how speech is framed visually via emoji, where the presentation and perception of oneself is constructed through creative visuality. Using an implicit frame analytical approach, Hu and colleagues (2014) surveyed and distinguished eight types of picture-framing sequences or clusters found on Instagram based on the following themes: friends, food, gadgets, captioned photos, pets, activities, selfies, and fashion. In all cases, the layout was a means to elicit a favorable impression or to obtain some goal. In another relevant study, Smith and Sanderson (2015) used Goffman's notion of self-presentation to examine the Instagram feeds of twenty-seven professional athletes. The researchers analyzed the use of photographs, accompanying captions, and hashtags to establish what the objectives of the athletes were and what general implications can be gleaned from them. The main finding was that, despite the conventional belief that men are traditionally framed with closer power headshots and women from a distance, in their personal Instagram feeds, both male and female athletes posted photos that displayed their full bodies, exuding a sense of empowerment.

It can be argued here that framing clinician–patient communications with emoji can achieve similar results, such as favorable impressions and a sense of patient empowerment. The layout of the emoji achieves this via episodic structure, highlighting the relevant events, situations, and so on that are relevant to the diagnostic situation at hand, attenuating any negative flow of meaning (as the Hu et al. study implies more generally).

The concept of image schema comes from conceptual metaphor theory, a model spearheaded by linguist George Lakoff (for example, Lakoff, 1979, 1987; Johnson 1987; Lakoff and Johnson 1980, 1999). As such, it is defined as a mental imagistic outline that guides the formation of an abstract concept. When we say "My mind is *full* of good memories," we are conceptualizing memory as a substance in a container (the brain). The container is an image schema that allows us to conceptualize and to frame abstractions in specific, understandable ways based on the experience of containers. It can be argued that an emoji is a kind of image schema that frames a concept visually. Consider, the orientation image schema of *up* versus *down*. This is derived from experiencing orientation in the real world, which then guides the framing of a host of concepts that are felt to implicate it in some imaginary way. Table 3.2 offers a few examples of how emoji realize this image schema representationally.

The range of image schemas is constrained by actual physical and affective experiences related to everyday events. Early work by Michael Reddy (1979) indicated that some are universal, since they translate common experiences, while others are more culture-specific. The container image schema noted earlier is seemingly universal, whereby mental states (feelings, ideas, concepts, etc.) are perceived to be substances that are put into linguistic containers (words, sentences, etc.), whose meanings are then extracted by listeners or readers, akin to taking substances or objects out of their containers.

Table 3.2 *Emoji as orientation image schemas*

Image schema	Frame	Emoji
Happiness is up	Reactions to a medical event: "My grandson is finally feeling up after a long bout with the flu."	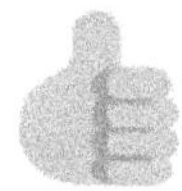 The thumbs-up gesture is a visual representation of the up-schema (depicting the actual gesture). It must always be kept in mind that this image schema is, as mentioned previously, culture-specific.
Sadness is down	Reactions to a disease: "I am feeling down, since I caught the flu."	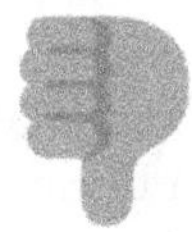 The thumbs-down represents the down-schema, again in visual-gestural suggestive form. Again, this emoji framing of the image schema is culture-specific.
More is up	Reactions to a symptom: "My fever was really high!"	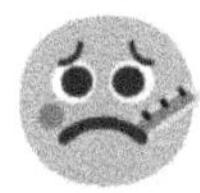 The thermometer emoji allows for a visualization of the more-is-up schema in an experienced-based way (given the familiarity most people have with thermometers).
Less is down	Reactions to a condition: "My energies are really down."	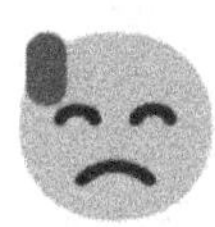 The downward dripping sweat and downward-turned mouth on this emoji render the less-is-down image schema suggestively.

Another one is the conduit image schema, which frames how we conceptualize the transmission of ideas, as if they were in a conduit ("Let me give you some advice," "I always pass on any new ideas to my students," and so on). From Reddy's analysis, the notion of discourse frames crystallized. There are many kinds of frames for talking about health that emoji permit (similar to the ones illustrated earlier); suffice it to say here that emoji-based clinician–patient healthcare communications allow for an image-schematic framing of medical information that allows patients to envision commonalities of experience and understanding with their healthcare practitioners. Emoji allow for a visual annotation of the reasons why certain things are felt to be connected, and in which ways they are connected. They also give coherence to specific topics, given their episodic structure (discussed further in Chapter 7).

A central motivation for using emoji in educational settings is the potential for tapping into students' hybrid literacy and its verbal–visual sign system (as discussed in Chapter 2). A second one is based on the fact, as just described, that emoji enfold unconscious image schemas that guide how students conceptualize and frame their ideas in digital communications. The semiotic modalities in image-schematic framing are embedded within it. One of these is iconicity, whereby the emoji stands for a referent through some form of resemblance. The smiley is, at a basic image-schematic level, an icon since it aims to portray a facial expression by an outline resemblance of the main features of the face that convey happiness. Emoji realizations of indexical image schemas, such as the orientation one discussed previously, are also intrinsic to the shape that emoji take – indexes are signs that stand for a referent by relating it (explicitly or implicitly) to other referents. Typically, though, iconicity and indexicality are intertwined. Consider the two-finger emoji indicating opposite directions shown in Figure 3.3.

At a primary level, the emoji embeds an iconic image schema, representing the hands and fingers via resemblance. But the different directions of the pointing fingers form an indexical opposition, right versus left. Finally, if intended to show where something is, such as in a public place, the two emoji can be used separately to indicate direction, which is a symbolic frame, since we need to know that they have been chosen, by convention, to constitute a particular type of directional sign.

The last comment requires a brief commentary here, since it emphasizes that emoji, like other sign structures, exhibit "oppositional structure," as it is commonly called in semiotics, that is, they are understood not in the absolute but rather in relation to other signs, a psychological phenomenon that Saussure (1916: 121–122) called *différence*. For example, in verbal language the minimal phonemic cues that make up words trigger meaning differences: "A linguistic system is a series of differences of sound combined with a series of

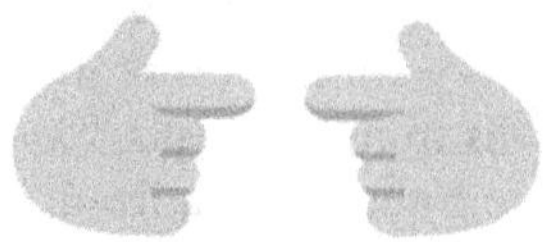

Figure 3.3 Pointing finger emoji

differences of ideas." It is *différence* that, arguably, activates critical thinking in understanding things and, thus, as a mechanism in learning. A simple example is the *différence* between the words *cat* and *rat*, which manifests itself in terms of the minimal sound contrast at the start of the words (*c* versus *r*). Now, the *différence* is distributed at other levels – by naming a type of animal as a *cat*, we have necessarily differentiated it conceptually from other animals, such as *rats*. So, the *différence* at this level becomes part of a system of oppositions, as they came to be known eventually (Ogden 1932), where animals called *cats* are differentiated from the other animals, perceived as *non-cats*. Now, having distinguished cats from non-cats bears cognitive consequences – by having the word *cat* in our mental lexicon we are predisposed to attend to the presence of this creature in the world as unique. Armed with that word, we start to perceive the existence of creatures that have physical affinities to *cats* – including whiskers, tails, and retractile claws, for instance. This suggests a larger category. In English, the name for that category is *feline*. Cultures stop their classificatory decision-making when they no longer see differentiations as useful or necessary. The process of opposition is not a conscious act, intuitively deepening one's understanding of an idea via its inclusion in a set of ideas, thus serving as a type of unconscious active learning.

Because of image-schematic and oppositional structure, emoji lend themselves as effective pedagogical devices, since they impel the learner to make comparisons and associations visually (without verbal cues), which is effective as part of learning (for instance, Danesi 2017). Work has shown that there is gradience between signs in semiotic opposition, which need not concern us here, since it would be beyond the present scope. As an illustrative example, in an opposition such as *white* versus *black*, various color concepts such as *gray*, *red*, and so on can be located between them, a fact that clearly has both referential and physical resonance – gradient colors are distributed on the light spectrum, while *white* and *black* are not, forming instead conceptual endpoints on a color scale. Similarly, the opposition *day* versus *night* is filled in with gradient concepts such as *twilight*, *dawn*, *noon*, and *afternoon*. This gradience is the likely source of nuanced thinking and, given its gradient variants, emoji may actually reveal or activate in the learner the fact that an idea exists not in the absolute but rather relative to other ideas.

A related concept to opposition is that of markedness, whereby one of the "poles" in an opposition is deemed to be the "expected" one and the other the "unexpected" or "derivative one." Markedness is a natural process of recognition that highlights the meaning of an idea. This is not only important to identification of ideas and their learning, it is also deeply rooted in, and reflective of, our social acculturation. A simple example of what this implies is an alarm device. We expect the device to be in an "off" mode in normal circumstances; when it goes "on" then we know that something is amiss. The "off" state is called the "unmarked" one and the "on" state, the "marked" one. Another way to describe the system is that the "off" mode indicates "absence of danger," while the "on" mode indicates "presence of danger." This absence-versus-presence opposition appears to be an underlying meta-opposition in sign systems. So, for example, in *day* versus *night*, *night* is typically conceived as being "absence of daylight," while *day* is rarely conceived analogously as being "absence of night time." In other words, *night* is "marked" conceptually with respect to *day*, which is perceived to be the "unmarked" concept in the opposition. Analogously, in the *happy*-versus-*sad* opposition related to the smiley, it can be argued that the happy face is the unmarked form, since we likely expect it to be the one used in digital messages as if by default. When the sad face is used, it bears a meaning that stands out, capturing our attention much more readily.

The gist of the foregoing discussion is that, while emoji are sign structures of a new and special kind, they still obey the laws of semiotics and conceptual framing. As picture words they correspond to the image-schematic intent of regular words, especially metaphors; as pictures, they are visible signs that allow for the framing of notions in holistic ways. To recall the ideas of Charles Morris (1938, 1946) here, signs such as emoji are subject to three main laws of semiosis: (1) syntactics, or the ability of signs to form assemblages to produce composite meanings; (2) semantics, or the relations that are forged between signs and their meanings, including oppositions and representational levels; and (3) pragmatics, or the discursive relations that are established between signs and their users, including how meaning is framed via signs. As a general insight, it can be suggested that as conceptual framing devices, emoji are a powerful way for learners to make sense of information, analyze concepts, and construct new knowledge relevant to their existing knowledge. The image-schematic framing of emoji leverages meaning-making in digital communication.

Emoji as Learning Tools

An emoji-based approach to education would involve the use of emoji that are actually used in everyday communications, especially those that can help concretize information. Given the many benefits that emoji use in clinician–practitioner interactions have been shown to bring about, their edusemiotic use in training healthcare professionals is a logical step, given that such training would arguably allow practitioners to gain a type of literacy that they would need in their clinical practices. Another reason is that the training itself would likely facilitate learning, as San-Martin et al. (2017) have emphasized: "in medical schools where a semiotic-based curriculum is offered, the empathetic orientation of medical students improves as a consequence of the acquisition and development of students' communication skills that are required in clinician–patient encounters."

Despite evidence supporting the importance of bringing emoji literacy into the classroom in general (Bhattacharya et al. 2019), it is also true that some practitioners remain largely skeptical about the efficacy and professionalism of using emoji in medicine. Among the reasons for this are: the potential to appear unprofessional, a lack of standardization of medical emoji, and platform and software variability, whereby a recipient might translate an emoji in such a way that it loses its intended meaning because of its platform-based form. However, as will be discussed and illustrated in the remainder of this book, such fears are relatively moot, given that emoji literacy constitutes simply a way to frame ideas in the Internet age. As the project carried out by Palaganas (Chapter 4) has shown, if exposed to emoji practically, practitioners tend to change their views favorably as they come to realize that the emoji system is nothing more than an informal mode of the pragmatic framing of ideas.

From a psychological standpoint, the incorporation of emoji in training formats of all kinds involves bimodal processing, which is arguably how learning can be optimized in various ways and situations. One of these is that they activate R-Mode and L-Mode stages both in tandem and in terms of a flow from the R-Mode to the L-Mode. This learning system involves the following features:

- Emoji allow the learner to become cognitively involved in a phase of learning within the cognitive space that the phase entails.
- Learners can be involved creatively in the learning space via allowance of their own creative use of emoji.

By reflecting on the whole event in blended visual and verbal ways, the learner assimilates the form-to-meaning relations that are inherent in a specific lesson or content.

As discussed, bimodality theory suggests that novel learning tasks require a high degree of creative involvement on the part of the learner – an R-Mode function; while reinforcement of learning and reflection on the structure and organization of the learned materials requires more formal involvement – an L-Mode function, in line with Vygotsky's (1961) suggestion that learners will demonstrate by their behavior when they have reached the point when the two modes become interdependent. The attainment of learning level will, of course, vary from student to student in terms of breadth (how much a particular individual is capable of learning something) and duration (the length of time the individual needs to grasp some learning task); but the attainment of each one will show up invariably, *for a particular student*, in appropriate behavior.

Emoji can be selected and used as general learning tools, given that they are not as constrained as more traditional verbal teaching tools might be, which assume sophisticated background knowledge. As such, emoji allow all kinds of students to: (1) grasp the meaning of the emoji via its presentation; (2) visualize the situation it presents; and then (3) induce them to conceptualize and explicate it in verbal terms. It is thus a type of pedagogical tool that lends itself to implicit learning and to the transference of this learning to more formal domains of knowledge.

Bimodality theory is consistent with the classic work in educational psychology and on mental development. In Jean Piaget's research, for instance (Piaget 1969), three stages are posited – sensory-motor, concrete operations, formal-logical thinking – that have become widely accepted as the primary cognitive milestones on the route to mental maturation. Piaget showed that humans progress from a sensory and concrete stage of understanding to a reflective and abstract one. Around the age of 2, children, according to Piaget's observations, start to develop symbolic abilities derived from mental images. As these become more dynamic, they prepare the child for more abstract thinking. Knowledge in the child thus emerges in terms of a direct relation to events in the immediate environment via the sensory apparatus and its ability to generate image schemas. Self-knowledge arises later. Piaget's theory has been called "genetic" – a term that he himself used to describe his approach. Clearly, the Piagetian stages are in line with the emoji-based model of bimodal teaching being proposed here – emoji evoke practical experiences via their image-schematic visuality, which corresponds to the sensory and concrete operations stage, leading to generalizations, which correspond to the reflective and abstract stages.

Let us consider the work of Lev S. Vygotsky (1961) more closely, given its relevance. Vygotsky proposed developmental stages that go from external (physical and social) actions toward internal cognitive constructions and interior speech, via the mind's ability to construct images of external reality. His definition of speech as a "microcosm of consciousness" is particularly reflective of this, constituting a kind of "symbolic modeling system" of such consciousness. The child engages in nonverbal symbolism (action, play, drawing, painting, music, etc.), which has its source in the R-Mode, and also engages with imaginative constructs (narratives, fables, dramatizations, etc.), which extend the R-Mode toward the L-Mode, and finally oral expression and creative thinking on the way to the development of abstract thought.

What makes emoji framing a powerful tool for educational purposes, as well as in sciences that depend on human interaction, such as healthcare, is that it activates mental visualization, which seems to be fundamental in how we grasp abstract concepts. Emoji are thus visible forms of image-schematic thinking, which will thus activate unconscious processes that favor comprehension of novel concepts.

Epilogue

Currently, emoji are being created and used in various healthcare communicative situations across the board. This suggests that healthcare professionals are coming to the awareness that emoji are effective in physician–patient interactions and, by extension, that the training of healthcare professionals should include emoji literacy, as Dr. Shuhan He emphasized to us during our interview with him. Moreover, as argued here, emoji are effective learning tools since they enfold all the laws of semiosis in compact, intuitive ways, which allow for the transference of understanding in more technical areas. As the late semiotician Umberto Eco (2010: 58) remarked, doctors should become more aware of the fact that semiosis and health are intertwined, and this is why "a homeopathic purification (according to the Greek medical tradition and to its connections with the Dionysian rites) depended on a discursive strategy through which language and other semiotic systems could produce prepositional attitudes which would make people believe or act in a certain way." This citation encapsulates the raison d'être of utilizing emoji for promoting well-being, and for their systematic use in healthcare communications. As J. F. Burnum (1993: 939) insightfully states: "contexts in which the sign appears shape the meaning of the sign and may change it altogether."

Saint Augustine of Hippo was among the first to argue that natural signs (such as symptoms) and mental states were connected intrinsically (see Markus 1957). Symptoms occur in reaction to altered bodily states; they have no intent in doing so. It is through our conventional sign systems, such as words and symbols, that we come to understand the meaning of the symptoms (on our own terms). As he put it in his *De Doctrina Christiana*: "A sign is a thing which causes us to think of something beyond the impression the thing itself makes upon the senses" (Vance 2010: 65). It is by "thinking beyond" impressions that we come to an understanding of what disease or well-being is. In effect, we cannot extricate symptomatology from how we understand it.

A sign selects what is considered at specific moments in time as important to be known and recalled from the infinite variety of impressions that we extract from the world. It imprints knowledge onto the brain in outline form, so as to filter out extraneous (meaningless) information. Although we create new signs to help us gain new knowledge and modify previous knowledge, by and large, we literally let our signs "do the thinking" for us, once we have acquired them in context. We are born into an already-fixed semiosphere, as the Estonian semiotician Yuri Lotman (1990) called it, that will largely determine how we view the world around us. This is the realm of signs and sign processes that guide human life. The biosphere sustains biological life on the basis of genetic information available to the species; by extension, the semiosphere sustains semiotic life (based on nongenetic information) through expressive, communicative, and representational activities, forming a kind of symbiotic partnership with the biosphere to shape human life and its evolution. But it is not a deterministic partnership. Humans have the capacity to redesign aspects of semiotic life and thus completely refashion the semiosphere. It remains to be seen how this partnership will evolve in the current digital semiosphere, or simply digisphere. At present, though, it would be ill advised to ignore a key sign system in the digisphere – the emoji one – given its key role within it.

Polish-American scholar Alfred Korzybski argued that human knowledge is limited by both the human nervous system and the languages and symbols humans have developed, implying that we can never have direct access to reality. As he famously put it (Korzybski 1933: 58): "A map is not the territory it represents, but, if correct, it has a similar structure to the territory, which accounts for its usefulness." Korzybski's clever example can be translated for the present purposes into "the emoji is not the thing for which it stands, but much more." Emoji have been an intrinsic part of the "digital maps" we have created in the digisphere, to extend the metaphor, reshaping the territory (the realm of meaning). McLuhan (1964) used a derivative metaphor, comparing language to the wheel as a means of navigating the territory: "Language does for intelligence what the wheel does for the feet and the body. It enables them to move from thing to thing with greater ease and speed and ever less involvement."

In sum, the use of emoji in healthcare situations and in training practitioners to be conversant in emoji speech will arguably make clinical interactions with patients much more effective. They can also speed up the collection of information in health-based situations where the patient might not be able to communicate well using verbal cues. However, problems exist that will need to be resolved according to specific situations, as is the case with everyday hybrid discourse, since emoji use is context-based and might differ across all kinds of social and psychological boundaries. Also, the degree of exactness between real sentiments or experience and emoji is still to be understood – an area that is receiving rather extensive attention within both the human cognitive sciences and artificial intelligence. A study in AI-based emoji sentiment analysis by Bale Chen (2023) has shown how AI can help assess the degree of fidelity between real sentiments and emoji representations. The key takeaway from his project was that emoji mark sentiment annotatively throughout their distribution in texts – a key finding that supports many of our own conclusions. If this is so, then clearly, emoji avoidance in healthcare and education may be unintentionally anachronistic and thus out of sync with how we communicate (and think) today.

4 A Mixed Methods Study

Prologue

The rationale for using emoji in clinician–patient communications and, by extension, in the training of healthcare professionals, was broached in the previous chapter. There are many relevant data sources that provide a wide range of empirically based insights into the reasons for emoji use in healthcare, including clinical shift phone texts, communication management platforms, patient charts with provider–patient texts, and informal team phone texts. However, studying these kinds of data is socially problematic, given the sensitive nature of patient information and provider–employer rights, all of which must be kept private. The need to protect such data and rights compelled one of the authors of this book, Janice Palaganas, to explore lower-stake ways to study the systematic use of emoji by healthcare professionals and to glean from this any educational implications for the training of practitioners.

Within these constraints, the present chapter presents the results of the Palaganas study involving participants in an online continuing education course that used an emoji-capable, text-based platform, offered through the Center for Medical Simulation in Boston, Massachusetts. The course was given in sessions at different times. The description that was posted for the course is as follows:

> Course Description. The course, *The Feedback Course*, is a 6-week online course designed to help practicing health professionals and health professions educators or leaders have effective feedback conversations with trainees and other team members. A 2-hour synchronous session occurs each of the six weeks. There is approximately an additional 3 hours of asynchronous work per week exclusively held within the Slack© application. The Slack workspaces have text interactions, some with manually entered emoji, as well as built-in emoji reaction options for each post. The participants for this course (approximately 12 to 20 per course) are practicing and experienced health professionals over 21 years of age that are interprofessional representing a range of health professions (e.g., physicians, nurses, physician assistants, paramedics, respiratory therapists, social workers, managers, researchers, educators, etc.), and international (approximately 60% are US-based with the other 40% a mixture of Europe, Australia, Asia, and the Middle East). Part of the course is receiving and giving frequent feedback from faculty and peers.

The registrants were practicing healthcare providers who were required to engage with each other through the platform. The study was designed and spearheaded by Palaganas, as mentioned, a professor at the Massachusetts General Hospital Institute of Health Professions and Lecturer at Harvard Medical School, together with a small team of researchers, including Dr. Temple Ratcliffe, who undertook a critical literature review of emoji use in the health professions. To assay the significance of the findings, two of the authors of this book (Palaganas and Petcoff) interviewed Dr. Shuhan He, whose work was discussed briefly in the previous chapter, and who is a leading expert on the use of emoji in healthcare practice at the patient-care level, as well as Dr. Neil Cohn, a leading researcher on the discourse features of emoji.

The methodology employed was qualitative mixed methods, which included the following main components:

(1) A questionnaire-survey designed to extract relevant information from the participants, including a demographic analysis of the emoji users (profession, gender, etc.) and their level of comfort in using the relevant platform (Slack).
(2) A Google form was prepared for each student with a screenshot of emoji uses.
(3) Interviews were conducted with focus groups, involving both structured and open-ended questions, as corroborative information for the overall findings. A discourse analysis of the data compiled from five of the sessions of the course was carried out.
(4) The questions posed to the practitioners at the start included the following:
    (a) When would you consider using emoji for healthcare-related issues?
    (b) Are there ideal instances for using them?
    (c) Are there any instances to avoid using them?
    (d) Why do you think health professionals choose to use emoji in a particular setting (online, asynchronous educational venues)?
    (e) What are the benefits (if any) of emoji use in these settings?
    (f) What concerns (if any) are there regarding emoji use in these settings?
    (g) How does emoji writing compare with other modes of professional communication? Do you feel that it is or is not professional?

As a pilot project, the aim was, overall, to determine how emoji use is perceived by healthcare professionals, how they use them (if at all), and the reasons for doing so. The results harbor implications for healthcare interactions and for the education of healthcare professionals more generally, which will be discussed more concretely in the next chapter.

Emoji use is seeping more and more into the healthcare professions, including clinically based communications practices, coworker texting, and patient–provider communications (Chapter 3). This has generated some angst and resistance among certain practitioners who may regard emoji as unprofessional.

Most hospital clinical shift phones, as well as patient communication systems, are mainly script character-only, despite the now routine use of emoji in other professions, such as business, education, and the law. Although the use of emoji is still not researched broadly in healthcare professions, there is no reason to believe that their use in this area as well will not produce the same pattern of positive results, especially in promoting congenial communications between practitioners and patients (Beißwenger and Pappert 2019). While there are still practitioners who might resist new media forms of communicating, the widening acceptance of emoji in common online platforms for both synchronous meetings (Zoom©, Microsoft Teams©) and asynchronous communications (Slack©) began during the COVID-19 pandemic (Hodges et al. 2020). Emoji availability on these platforms made their use increasingly acceptable, as a way to indicate participant engagement; degree of interest in, and association with, the topic discussed; and negotiating and establishing interpersonal relationships.

The Palaganas project was approved in 2018 by the Institutional Review Board and the Partners Healthcare Human Research Office Institutional Review Boards (Protocol ID: 2018P001533). In order to allow the online conversations to flow freely and to prevent injecting any bias into emoji usage, the Slack conversations were analyzed retrospectively, after being conducted prospectively. The six sessions were held in March 2019, January 2020, September 2020, March 2021, October 2021, and March 2022, after which a discourse analysis of the Slack conversations in all the courses was carried out. To ensure anonymity the following general instruction was used:

> Please fill out this questionnaire and answer each question as best as you can. All questions are optional. Please do not include your name. Thank you so much for your time and thoughts. If you have any trouble accessing or completing this survey, please email us.

In addition to a general consent form that the participants completed prior to the study, permission to use the results was asked at various stages of the project. The general template used in this case is shown next:

> Permission to Publish Question … Responses: Your responses will be deidentified and we will be thematically analyzing your typed responses. We may feel that your snapshot is the best example of what we find. If this is the case, we would deidentify your message. This being said, your typed responses, while not identifiable to the public, they may be identified by other course participants by the snapshot. For this reason, each question will additionally ask if you do not consent to the publication of each particular snapshot and your response – both will be publicly deidentified but may be identified by others in the course. Do you approve the use of the above snapshot deidentified for future publications?

Participants

No remunerative incentives for participation were offered. The participant demographics were elicited via the last section of the questionnaire.

What is your profession?
Your answer:

What is your country of residence?
Your answer:

What is the ethnic or global culture with which you identify?
Your answer:

What is your year (only) of birth?
Your answer:

What is your identified gender?
Your answer:

The numerical breakdown of each session group was:

March 2019:	$N = 21$
January 2020:	$N = 25$
September 2020:	$N = 13$
March 2021:	$N = 13$
October 2021:	$N = 10$
March 2022:	$N = 11$
Total:	$N = 93$

The demographic variables were mapped against actual emoji use and in relation to individual perceptions of such use. The data were collected from each of the course session participants through the Slack platform. Additionally, two focus groups were selected from the March 2021 participants, so as to be able to evaluate the results more concretely. The breakdown of the participants is given in Table 4.1.

Table 4.1 *March 2021 group demographics*

Participant	Gender	Age	Discipline	Specialty	Geography
P1	M	40–50	Physician	Anesthesiology	Switzerland
P2	F	50–60	Nurse	Anesthesiology	USA
P3	F	40–50	Nurse	Maternal/Child Nursing	USA
P4	F	20–30	Nurse	Nurse Practitioner	USA
P5	M	30–40	Physician	Anesthesiology	Germany

Participant	Gender	Age	Discipline	Specialty	Geography
P6	F	20–30	Social Work	Social Work	Canada
P7	M	30–40	Administrator	Healthcare Admin	USA
P8	F	50–60	Nurse	Psychiatry	Germany
P9	F	20–30	Nurse	Pediatric Emergency	UK
P10	M	30–40	Emergency Services	Critical Care Transport	USA
P11	F	30–40	Educator/Researcher	Research (Sim)	USA
P12	F	20–30	Physician	Anesthesiology	USA
P13	F	40–50	Nurse	Perianesthesia/Critical Care	USA

Aims and Methods

The data were collected mainly via a personalized survey in which emoji uses were included and for which opinions were elicited, by both the senders and the receivers (discussed later in this chapter). The main goal was to explore the reasons healthcare professionals used (or did not use) emoji in their online Slack interactions, and what role semiotic and discourse functions emoji play in such interactions (if any). The aims of the study were, in effect, to address questions such as the following.

Who (of the Professionals) Would Use Emoji Regularly in Digital Communications?

The aim here was to match emoji use against variables such as profession, geography, age, and self-identified gender. For this reason, we used actual text messages containing emoji in Slack conversations and asked both the senders and the receivers questions about their use. This allowed for a retrospective descriptive analysis, mapping emoji use against the relevant demographic variables. The focus groups allowed for a face-to-face discussion regarding use patterns and comfort level with the use of emoji and with new technologies in general. The relevant questionnaire part is shown next.

How would you describe your comfort with Slack?

- I was not comfortable with Slack.
- I was somewhat comfortable with Slack.
- I was comfortable with Slack.
- I was extremely comfortable with Slack.

How would you describe your comfort with technology overall?

- I am not comfortable with technology.
- I am somewhat comfortable with technology.

- I am comfortable with technology.
- I am extremely comfortable with technology.

How would you describe your typical comfort level with a new phone app?

- Typically, I am not comfortable with a new phone app.
- Typically, I am somewhat comfortable with a new phone app.
- Typically, I am comfortable with a new phone app.
- Typically, I am extremely comfortable with a new phone app

How often are you on social media?

- Everyday
- Every other day
- Once a week
- Rarely

Do you use emoji in your daily communications? If yes, when?
Your answer:

Do you use emoticon reactions in your daily communications? If yes, when?
Your answer:

What Emoji Are Used?

Another aim of the study was to assess if certain types of emoji are used more frequently by healthcare professionals than the general population and if such usage aligns with daily social uses or differs according to profession. To answer this question, we performed a retrospective descriptive analysis of emoji types, comparing our findings to general emoji use, that is, to uses outside of the healthcare context, and by interviewing our two experts.

When Are Emoji Used?

Another objective of the project was to determine whether or not there were particular discourse or thematic situations when emoji were used or not used. The general findings in this area were a topic of discussion with the March 2021 focus group, which revolved around the question: When would you consider using emoji?

When Is It Appropriate and Inappropriate to Use Emoji?

This is a version of the previous question, aiming to ascertain more concretely if the healthcare professionals felt that emoji were appropriate or inappropriate in specific situations of interaction. For this question, the survey, interview, and focus group were enlisted to answer related aspects. The relevant questions used on the survey form were the following:

Why do health professional choose to use emoji in this setting (online, asynchronous educational)?
Your answer:

What are the benefits of using emoji in these settings?
Your answer:

What concerns (if any) are there regarding emoji use in these settings?
Your answer:

Referring to the previous question, how does this compare to use in other professional/personal communication?
Your answer:

Do you feel that emoji use in these settings is or isn't professional? Why or why not?
Your answer:

Do you use emoji in your clinical practice communications? Why or why not?
Your answer:

How do you think culture plays a role in emoji use? Please specify which type of culture you believe influences use (e.g., ethic, professional, organizational, generation, gender)?
Your answer:

How Are Emoji Used (That Is, in What Context)?
A major focus of interest is how emoji are used in, or constrained by, contextual aspects. Data on this area can inform ways to integrate healthcare literacy education with other types of literacy, such as the kind described in Chapter 2. Central to this question is how to train professionals to use emoji, so as to avert miscommunications.

Why Are Emoji Used (That Is, Individual Stated Reason for Use)?
To triangulate the data and check for researcher bias, we surveyed and conducted focus groups with the March 2021 cohort (as mentioned), so as to determine what the perceived reasons might be for using emoji. The specific questions used were: Why did you use this emoji? Why do health professionals choose to use emoji in this setting (online, asynchronous educational)?

Findings and Analyses

As mentioned, the findings were collected from Slack conversations, the focus groups, and follow-up questions based on the online conversations. These were then subjected to five types of analyses: (1) descriptive frequency analysis, (2) discourse analysis, (3) overall thematic analysis, (4) focus group specific thematic analysis, and (5) an interview thematic analysis.

To gather data on the actual conversations, the questionnaire contained relevant questions that both the senders and the receivers were required to answer. Examples of actual texts that were found on the Slack platform include:

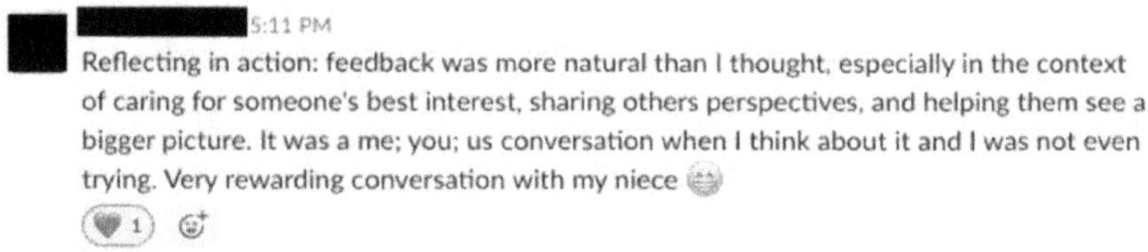

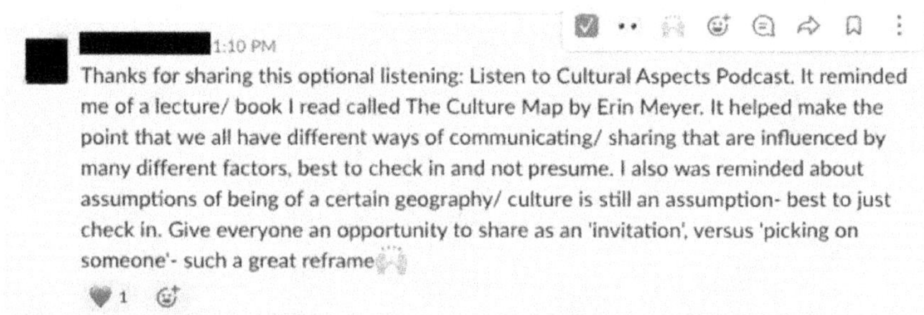

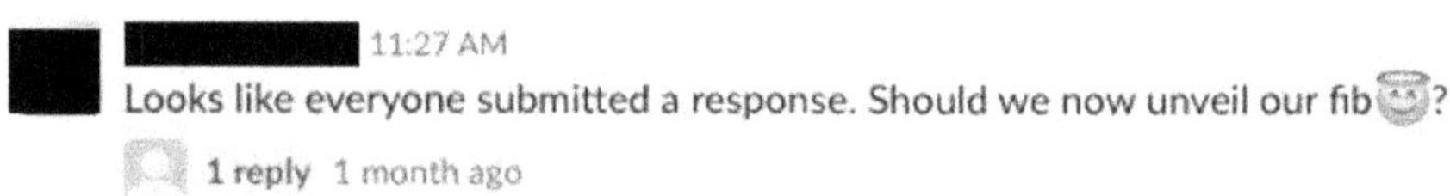

The senders and receivers of these texts were asked the same questions separately.

> The next few questions contain snapshots of your conversations in which you used emoji and/or emoji reactions. For each question, please review the snapshot. For additional context, a link to the actual Slack conversation is provided. For the purpose of this survey, an emoji is any picture character that you include in your text messages. Emoji reactions are the likes under each post.
>
> Why do you think you reacted to this message the way you did?
> Your answer:
>
> Why did you choose the emoji or emoticon you used?
> Your answer:

In all cases, the participants were given a link to see each message in context and to review the whole message thread. The responses to the questions were tabulated. They are discussed in different sections in the remainder of this chapter.

Descriptive Frequency Analysis

In order to correlate emoji type and frequency of use to profession, geography, age, and self-identified gender, we used a descriptive content frequency analysis of the Slack conversations. The relevant demographic data were collected using REDCap (Research Electronic Data Capture) (Harris et al. 2019) at the beginning of the course. We exported the intact html of all publicly posted conversations to the Slack site, consisting of six channels and conversation threads that typically focused on a topic or purpose saved on a secure partner's Dropbox file. Only the principal investigator (Palaganas) had access to the file. There was also: (1) one channel for general conversations among members of the course; (2) two or more small group channels (consisting of groups who generally worked together during the course); and (3) three or more specific topic channels (for feedback on cultural considerations, on the nature of the clinical environment, on the feedback itself, etc.). All conversations were then deidentified by the principal investigator, logged, coded for reference, and uploaded as screenshots to Dedoose (a qualitative data analysis software), so as to preserve the original Slack emoji image, which may have otherwise been altered or translated between platforms. The deidentified data was password-protected and only accessed by the principal investigator and one other researcher.

An analysis of frequency of usage and type of emoji used according to demographic variables was carried out and checked by comparison to the findings within the research team. Any discrepancy was rerun separately until a consensus was reached. As it turned out, the highest use of emoji occurred in the January 2021 session. The frequency chart in Figure 4.1 presents a summary.

The fact that the January group used emoji more than the others might seem peculiar, suggesting that emoji use may be related to a kind of pathetic fallacy, whereby meteorological and emotional climate become intertwined. While this may seem farfetched, it is certainly worth investigating further, since it could be matched against usage patterns in geographic areas that have a colder climate versus those by users who live in moderate or warm zones.

Another finding from the REDCap analysis allowed us to correlate emoji users to profession. As the graph in Figure 4.2 shows, the nurses in our sample used emoji more than the others, with physicians coming in just behind.

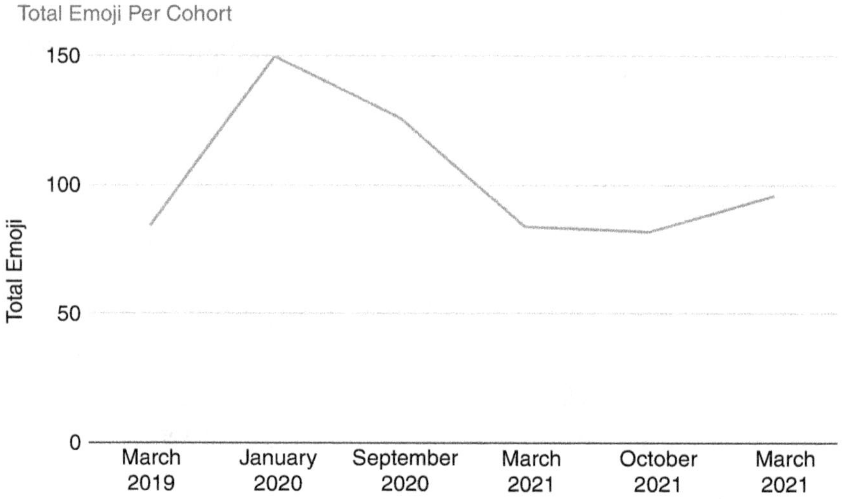

Figure 4.1 Frequency of emoji use per cohort

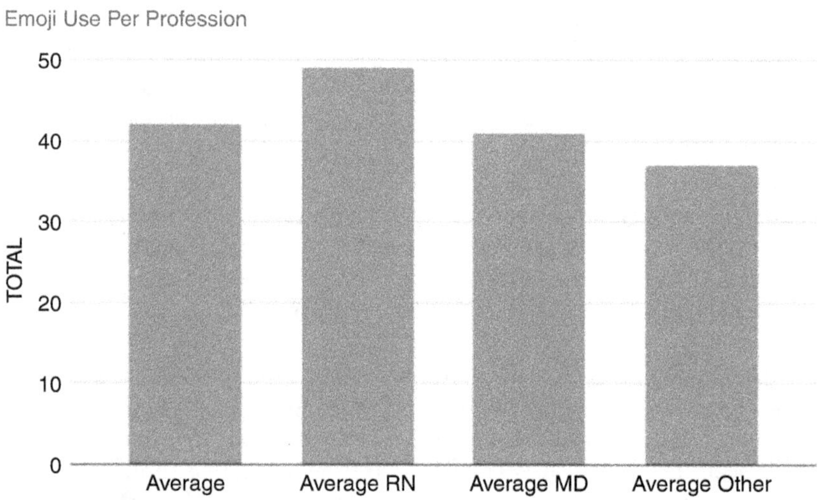

Figure 4.2 Frequency of emoji use per profession

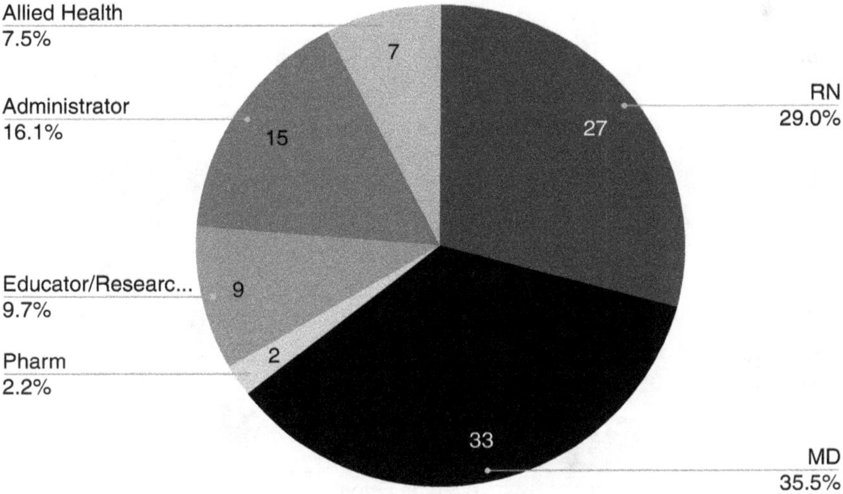

Figure 4.3 Participants according to profession

One reason for this was that the number of nurses enrolled in the course was second only to the number of doctors. All other categories were much smaller, as can be seen in Figure 4.3.

Another likely reason might relate to emoji use in general, which indicates that people in professions and jobs that involve sentiment and empathy, such as teachers and nurses, are more likely to use messages with high emotivity, as various studies suggest. For example, Marder et al. (2020) found that emoji usage by university instructors, who were mainly female in the sample, increased perceived warmth but did not impugn perceptions of competence, affecting student evaluation and task behavior positively. Erica Dhawan (2021), a nurse manager, similarly found that emoji use among nurses provided emotive texture and context to digital communications, even though ambiguities in meaning emerged.

Since the nursing participants in our study were primarily female, it also comes as little surprise that the women in the group were the highest users of emoji.

Female: 71%	($N = 66$)
Male: 29%	($N = 27$)
Other: 0%	($N = 0$)

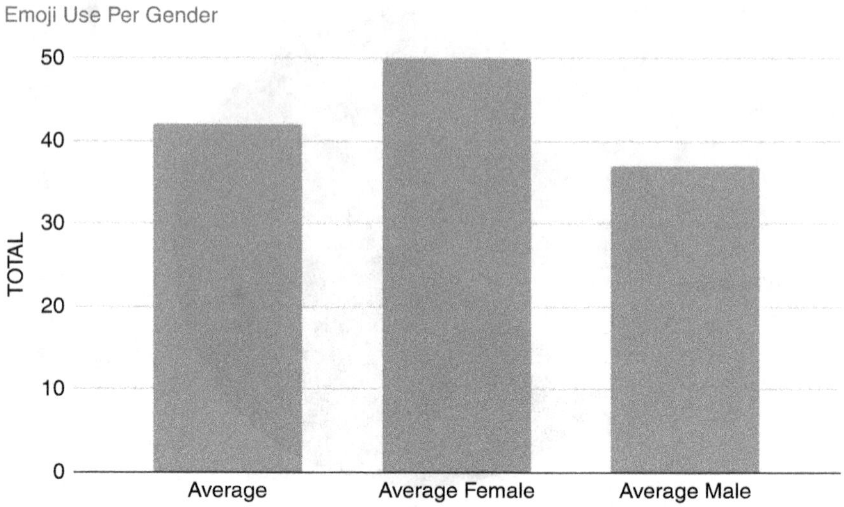

Figure 4.4 Frequency of emoji use per gender

Figure 4.4 indicates the frequency pattern according to gender.

This finding also correlates with more general findings, as mentioned, that have found that women use emoji more than men and generally have a better knowledge of their different meanings (for example, Butterworth et al. 2019).

The age distribution of our participant sample is given in Figure 4.5 – note that the largest category was the 30–40 one:

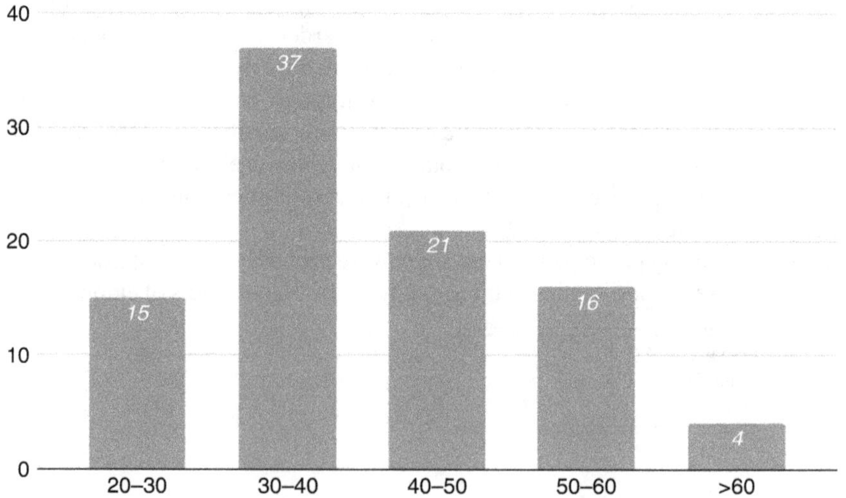

Figure 4.5 Participants according to age

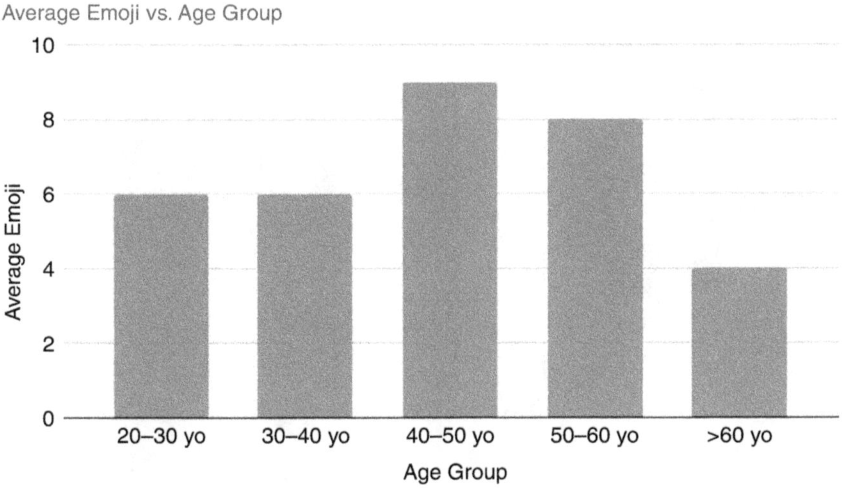

Figure 4.6 Frequency of emoji use per age group

Surprisingly, it was found that that emoji use according to age was higher in the 40–60 age range (Figure 4.6).

Studies now show that age-based differences have in fact emerged with regard to emoji usage, and that some of those that emerged as more commonly used in the Palaganas study are actually now discarded by the younger generations (as of 2022). These included (see Table 4.2) the thumbs-up, red heart, OK hand, checkmark, loud crying face, and the grimacing face. It is interesting to note that the "mid age" groups were frequent users, suggesting that the "older emoji" are now part of the emoji competence of "older users," and thus that emoji usage is evolving from one generation to the next, much like words in verbal language.

The geographic distribution of the study participants is shown in Figure 4.7.

As it turned out, participants from North America and Australia used emoji more than participants from other countries (Figure 4.8).

This finding correlates with the general literature on emoji usage. However, research is also showing that emoji use is diffusing in ever-changing ways, so that it is difficult to pinpoint which countries have the highest and which the lowest users. Moreover, each country seems to favor various emoji types, which may reveal some cultural motivation or specific socially based communicative reason for use, which need not concern us here. One factor that may be at play, but is not investigated by this particular study, is culturally based differences in emoji meanings that would inevitably guide user choice. This would, however, have bearing upon the teaching of emoji literacy. Consider a hypothetical situation, whereby a native English-speaking doctor from the

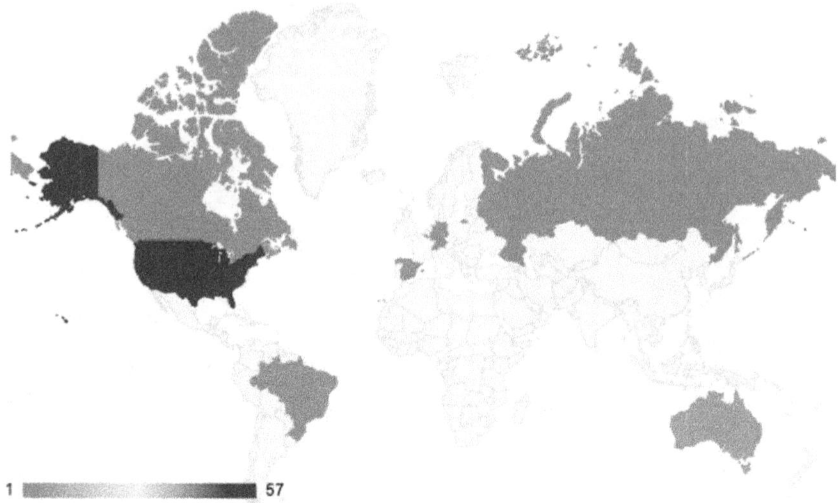

USA	Canada	Middle East	AUS	UK	Brazil	Belgium	Spain	Barbados	Germany	Switzerland	Russia
57	3	8	8	6	4	2	2	1	3	1	1

Figure 4.7 Participants according to geography

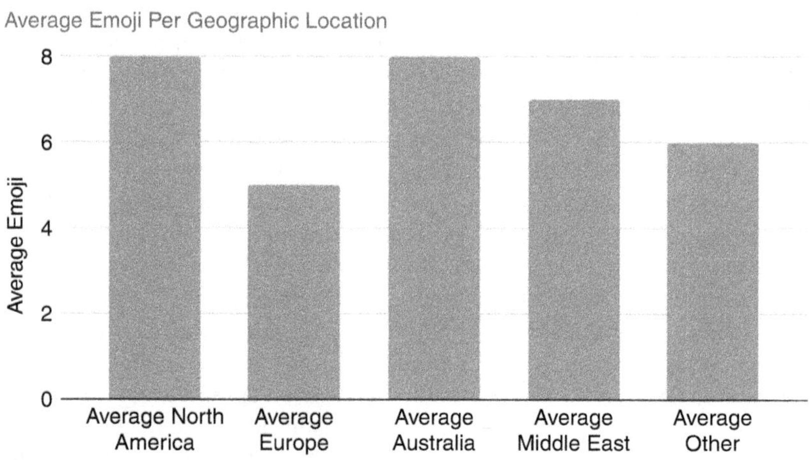

Figure 4.8 Emoji use per geographic location

United States writes a text message to several colleagues regarding an upcoming medical conference. In it, she uses the OK gesture 👌, without realizing that it could offend interlocutors in different countries, including receivers of her message in Iraq, Iran, and Greece, who might interpret it as an obscene gesture.

Table 4.2 *Types of emoji used*

✅	190	👀	10	👋	5	💪	2
👍	103	😮	9	🤔	4	🍿	1
😆	48	🙂	9	😍	3	🇦🇺	1
❤️	42	😅	9	😠	3	💡	1
💯	32	😁	9	😬	3	🦮	1
😂	28	🤦	8	👏	3		
🙌	26	🎉	8	🤷‍♀️	3		
🙏	12	🤣	8	🙁	3		
🙋‍♀️	12	😃	6	😑	2		
😌	11	🙄	5	🤩	2		

Summarily, the actual types that were found to characterize the online conversations and their frequencies are charted in Table 4.2.

Even a cursory perusal of the results indicates that: (1) the most frequent types used were the those listed by Unicode as the more widely used emoji across the world (mainly facial and gestural), and (2) the distribution according to participant variables was also consistent with the Unicode data regarding who uses emoji more than others and where they are used (discussed later in this chapter).

Discourse Analysis

In order to understand the factors influencing when and how emoji are used, we carried out a generic discourse analysis of the Slack content from all course sessions, in line with similar analyses found in the relevant literature

(Chapter 1). There were over 5,200 messages from ninety-three participants. To ensure confidentiality and privacy, all participants were informed in advance of the research and their consent was ascertained in writing (as mentioned). The Slack Application Program Interface was used to collect the messages, which were then exported as a computerized system validation file, securely stored in a partner's password-protected Dropbox file. The messages were organized chronologically, deidentified, and labeled with a respective research participant number. Each message was coded according to type of emoji, demographics, and content topic, such as assignments, inquiries, social interactions, stories, and requests for feedback. A codebook was generated based on this information, created by two researchers on the team who met weekly to review the coding data and to reach a consensus so as to delineate the actual types of codes and the codebook required.

The analysis revealed several key themes and patterns, which can be summarized as follows:

(1) The participants employed positive and inclusive language that served as a form of communicative reassurance for the entire community, which included statements such as "caring for someone's best interest," "sharing others' perspectives," "we all have different ways of communicating/sharing that are influenced by many different factors." The smiley emoji encapsulated the main sentiment, distributed semantically across the messages.
(2) Across demographics, emoji were mostly used in messages that revolved around subjective information, such as a personal story, as exemplified in one of the messages: "Very rewarding conversation with my niece." The same smiley face emoji provided the relevant visual annotation to this content.
(3) A coding of the text messages according to user revealed that there were clear conversation "leaders" and "cheerleaders" in each session cohort, whereby specific individuals would dominate conversations, and the others (cheerleaders, so to speak) would follow the leader's prompts with supportive comments, utilizing positive emoji in a distributive manner.
(4) The leaders used less emoji and replied via script to most comments. They tended to be physicians, except in one cohort where the leader was an administrator.
(5) Cheerleaders tended to be nurses, except in two cohorts, where one was a simulationist and another a physical therapist.

Survey Thematic Analysis

The survey was administered using Google forms and took approximately twenty-five minutes to complete. It included both multiple-choice and open-ended questions. It consisted of five sections: demographics, comfort with technology, user of emoji/emoji reactions, receiver of emoji/emoji reaction, emoji and health professions education. The kinds of questions used are provided earlier in this chapter. The sections "user of emoji/emoji reactions" and "receiver of emoji/emoji reaction" were personalized by including a screenshot of the communication where the emoji were used. To best answer the open-text questions following the screenshot, a link to the entire communication thread where the screenshot was taken was also provided. This allowed a participant to explore the full context in which the emoji was used. The questions following each screenshot asked why the emoji was chosen and how one felt about using it. Respondents were able to change answers on the survey but prevented from submitting more than one survey. Because the surveys were personalized, IP addresses were not collected. The survey link was open over a two-week period after the conclusion of the course.

The data were cleaned, compiled, and analyzed using Dedoose version 9.0.17. A thematic analysis was performed (Braun and Clarke 2012) on the user of emoji/emoji reactions, receiver of emoji/emoji reaction, and emoji and health professions education sections. The team researchers had familiarized themselves with the data independently, coded each response, generated themes inductively for each section, and iteratively reviewed the themes together, so as to come to a consensus. Additionally, the data were mapped against the demographic data for comparison purposes. When analyzing the "user of emoji/emoji reactions" and "receiver of emoji/emoji reaction" sections, the researchers took journal notes on their initial perceptions prior to reading the survey responses. These were discussed during the review sessions. Furthermore, user data was compared with receiver data for relevant data points. A response rate of 100 percent for each question was achieved. Only one participant reentered the site to revise their survey.

The results are listed below:

(1) The differences noted as per profession, country of residence, age, self-identified gender, comfort with technology, and daily use of emoji were discussed earlier in the descriptive frequency analysis section.
(2) The two main reasons identified by the participants for using emoji are: (a) it felt psychologically safe to do so in the situation provided by the course, and (b) it was a way to express emotions, such as anxiety, uncertainty, and even playfulness, effectively and economically. When asked specifically why they chose a particular emoji, the main reasons included: (a) the emoji best captured how the participant was feeling and (b) it was the most accessible technically.
(3) The receivers of the emoji-containing messages were asked why they thought certain emoji were used by the senders. The main explication given was to show engagement. Other responses varied, including the need to show

empathy with the sender, agreement ("I agreed with the content, I wanted to emphasize what was stated"), emotional support ("I wanted to encourage the other person, I wanted to show understanding and empathy"), and affinity with the sender ("I wanted to seem more friendly"). Interestingly, when asked specifically why they thought a particular emoji was chosen by the sender, six participants admitted bluntly "I don't know why."

(4) The senders were asked the same questions as the receivers, and they too replied in a similar way, emphasizing that they wanted to be validated and reassured. One participant even stated that they felt a need to establish a "human connection."

(5) As to the use of emoji in healthcare professions, there emerged a lack of consensus, with a clear dichotomy between those who felt that emoji use was professional and those who did not. Supporters mentioned that it helped convey nonverbal cues, allowing for more concrete interactions, while strengthening the phatic bonds between interlocutors. Opponents were concerned about the possibility of miscommunication, which might arise from accidentally selecting the wrong emoji. One participant stated that they were concerned about an overuse of emoji, since it would dilute the emotive power of using emoji.

(6) When asked about emoji in everyday communication, the younger participants said that they were more likely to use them.

(7) A major obstacle to adopting emoji was identified as the institutional culture in which one worked – that is, it would be anomalous to use emoji if their institution or organization did not.

Focus Group Thematic Analysis

In order to gain a fuller perspective on who used emoji, as well as when and why, two focus groups were formed from the March 2021 cohort. The participants were interviewed by two team researchers using an interview guide, conducted on Zoom (Partners Zoom Video Communications). The number of participants in each group was limited to five, as per standard practice in this domain of research (Lobe et al. 2020). The sessions were video recorded, transcribed using Zoom audio transcription, reviewed, deidentified, and edited for accuracy. They were then uploaded to Dedoose (Version 9.0) for thematic analysis.

The analysis involved several phases (Braun and Clarke 2012; Kiger and Varpio 2020). First, the team researchers familiarized themselves with the transcripts by reading them multiple times, paying attention to content, tone, and other relevant discourse and semiotic features. Second, each independently reviewed the first transcript, from which initial descriptive codes were generated (Saldaña 2020). The researchers then met to discuss the codes and to review and update the codebook, so as to ensure consensus prior to coding the second transcript. Coding continued iteratively until no new codes were identified as relevant. Third, the researchers independently searched for themes. Fourth, they reviewed these themes together as a group, mapping them to the data and discussing them with each other. Fifth, the themes were finally defined and established collaboratively. The five major themes that emerged are the following (encapsulated by the italicized comments):

(1) *Emoji made me want to engage.* Most of the participants felt that the use of emoji increased engagement and enhanced communication in the specific online learning environment in which the messages were created, pointing out that emoji use leveraged and attenuated the professional–personal dichotomy by providing a more informal mode of contact that bridged the social gap that tended to emerge in professional interactions. Following are relevant comments by the participants (P = participant number):

> "For me it was a form of validation from the group … whoever gave [a] thumbs up or things like that was a way for me to say okay, they understand me and I'm part of the group. So it engaged me to pursue and to go further" (P6).

> "I felt that maybe sometimes people didn't have enough time to express up a written statement on what they thought my post was about or what I was trying to say so, a quick thumbs up or some type of smiley face or reaction like that was validating for any point that I tried to make. And it also just helped me to feel more engaged" (P7).

> "We are socialized to be different in the professional setting so we all, most of us, try not to show our personal side too much at work or in these settings until you find a friend at work. The emoji breaks down that line and it opens up a more friendly connection" (P1).

(2) *It depends on my relationship with you.* Most of the participants felt that the use or avoidance of emoji was dependent on the type of social relationships that existed between interlocutors, rather than on professional roles. The degree of perceived social closeness in an interaction influenced emoji use. Following are two relevant comments:

> "I haven't thought of it as in terms of the discipline. More so I agree, like the relationship, you know it's the people that I am closer with that probably more so consider closer to friends or friends that I would get emojis from and might hardly ever get them from someone that's higher in the hierarchy and in a professional way or in a non-professional way" (P10).

> "That makes me think that maybe it's not completely hierarchy related, it is definitely yes, but maybe it's just relationship related" (P1).

(3) *You might not think it is professional, but I think it's fine.* There was a lack of consensus on the use of emoji in professional healthcare-related settings; that is, some were uncertain about whether or not the use of emoji diminished the perception of professionalism. Following are relevant comments:

> "I definitely would never use emoji on my work phones. It allows it, they are regular iPhones, but I just would never … it would just be unprofessional for me personally. I just don't do that" (P3).

> "We have to get with the times. It's natural to use it and I don't see a problem with it, so long as it is not a report about a patient" (P6).

> "However, I think … to just give a blanket answer … I think, less is definitely more, and there are very few emojis that I would actually share in any professional context, whether healthcare related or non-healthcare related" (P7).

> "Texting in general is such a thin platform. Like I sometimes don't know if someone is smiling or not. And at work, I'd want to know if something is bad or good, so I'd want that smiley face" (P4).

> "There are so many things that could go wrong using any kind of emoji. People might misinterpret things and the repercussions at work are much greater than in a social climate" (P12).

(4) *Some are acceptable in general, and some are definitely not.* There was full agreement that certain emoji are more acceptable than others in healthcare communications and could be used without danger of miscommunication or uncertain meaning. These included: the smiley face, the thumbs up, the arm strength, the applause, and the hand clap emoji. The emoji identified as problematic included: the fruit or vegetable, flushed face, and heart emoji. When clarity about patient care is critical and when one is not sure about the relationship with an interlocutor or with regard to the organizational culture, then emoji should be avoided. Following are two relevant comments:

> "Well, I think you have to be a little bit careful with the heart, one I use that as an example, at the beginning, because it felt warm to me, but I think it definitely, like what was just brought out, could be misinterpreted as something else and be very unprofessional" (P3).

> "Yeah well my opinion on that is don't use emojis when you're talking about the patients" (P8).

(5) *When our leader used it, I knew it was fine.* The implicit group leader dynamic (discussed earlier) provided the implicit rules for how and when to use emoji (or not). If a leader used them, the other members interpreted that as a signal that "it is okay to use them." If one replaces the notion

of leader with organization, the pattern of responses can be generalized. Following are relevant comments:

> "I think it might be different for different organizations … so I would I would … be wanting to watch and see how people were using them before I actually started using them more so I really think it has to do with your culture your organization and where you're working" (P3).

> "For example, in Teams, we have the thumbs up for agree, but we don't have a thumb down emoji, so we define the smiley which is looking sad as 'I cannot help' … and so I can just look into the emojis and go with a with a cursor and then I see who gave this emoji and I know okay 20 students are not able to do the course or can … and this is why we defined what is meant for which response" (P8).

> "In this course, when the instructor used it, I knew that I could use it, too. I liked that" (P7).

Interviews Thematic Analysis

To maximize the reliability and validity of our findings, an additional step was taken by interviewing a communications expert in emoji use (Dr. Cohn) and an expert in emoji use within healthcare (Dr. He). Scheduling of the interviews served as consent to participate freely. Each interview began with a general discussion of the study findings in their fields, after which the focus was put on the implications for the potential use of emoji in healthcare communications and education. The interviews were transcribed and coded for insights. Both experts anticipated that emoji will gradually enter medical and healthcare communications systematically, providing more options for effective expression over traditional text, especially in areas such as pediatrics, disabilities, psychiatry, and the like (see https://Medicalemoji.org). Both stressed that healthcare professionals can no longer resist trends in general communications and would thus be well advised to become fluent in what has been called hybrid literacy here.

It was pointed out that among the relevant additions to the emoji lexicon was the 2018 anatomical brain emoji, although not created specifically for healthcare use, and the anatomical heart and organ emoji, which were earmarked instead for medical use. Relevantly, the Wong-Baker FACES Pain Rating Scale, which prefigures emoji, has been widely used and accepted in healthcare situations since 1983, with numerous studies having come forth to document its efficacy. An issue identified by our experts was that healthcare is a science-based field where adoption most frequently stems from evidence-based reasoning. Hopefully, the findings of studies such as the one here, the experts agreed, might go a long way to establishing hybrid literacy as a viable option for communications in the healthcare world and as a basis for educational practices within that world (training practitioners in emoji literacy for specific healthcare motives).

Discussion

The findings of the project revealed a number of outcomes that suggest some preliminary answers as to who, what, when, how, and why emoji are used in the healthcare world. These are summarized in what follows.

Who Uses Emoji in Their Text-Based Communications?

As the study found, emoji are used by practitioners of all ages, demographics, and cultural backgrounds, in virtually the same way and within the same frequency ranges as the general public. Differences according to geography, age, or gender variables were predictable. The ninety-three participants over four years (2019–2022) employed 622 emoji in total and, as discussed earlier, it was found that 40–60-year-olds used more emoji than younger and older populations. It was also found that women used emoji more than men. Such findings align with the research outside of the healthcare context.

In effect, the perception of emoji use in the study sample did not differ significantly from the general perception of such use. Even though the study was based on a relatively small sample, there is no reason to believe that it does not harbor more general implications with respect to healthcare communications. Interestingly, the common assumption that emoji use is more frequent among younger generations was not supported by our study. While the participants themselves identified the younger members as the ones more likely to use emoji, the data did not bear this out, suggesting that at present emoji use has penetrated all age categories – age is seemingly not a factor influencing emoji use in the healthcare world. This does not preclude, however, the possibility that emoji meanings will vary according to age category, as discussed, with some emoji, like the heart, now marked as anachronistic by younger people (An et al. 2018).

What Emoji Are Used?

The findings suggest the kinds of emoji used by healthcare professionals are specialized as to meaning. For example, the red heart emoji has different, more specific medical meanings in healthcare communications that do not apply outside. This attenuates the possibility for the kinds of ambiguity, misinterpretations, and cultural-coding that have beset emoji usage globally. These outside factors may, nonetheless, influence the use of emoji in healthcare situations. Glikson and colleagues (2018) found that smileys do not necessarily increase perceptions of warmth (as they were designed to do) and in various workplaces they may even produce the opposite effect.

When Are Emoji Used?

Emoji are used in a wide range of contexts and situations to convey various discursive and semiotic functions. The participants were generally aware of this fact and favorable toward emoji use, with some exceptions (as mentioned earlier), including their use in communications where patient care is critical, when one is not sure of one's relationship with the interlocutor, and when usage is not prescribed by the relevant organizational culture in which the professionals find themselves. Some saw emoji as a psychologically safe way of expressing emotional states or moods, which might seem inappropriate with words. They indicated that interactions with a friendly interlocutor would make emoji use feel more appropriate, as it would if a leader of the community used emoji – that is, in situations where people are more likely to engage openly in dialogue, ask questions, and share thoughts willingly. We did not specifically explore psychological safety in our study, but it did come out suggestively (as discussed).

A pertinent finding of the study was that practitioner-based emoji use, while specialized for medical purposes, nonetheless is in line with its use by the global population, as witnessed especially by the fact that the main types of emoji used were the facial ones. It would seem that the primary use of emoji is to project subjectivity onto the written text via facial expressions in image-schematic form. As such, emoji provide a schematic picture of an inner thought, idea, emotion, or opinion. This differentiates them from traditional pictographs or ideographs per se, which are visual signs standing for an array of referents that correspond to verbalized concepts. Emoji are part of a communicative system designed to allow for the conveyance of subjectivity. The same conclusion was reached by Grosz and colleagues (2023), who put it as follows:

> We propose that there is a use of face emoji in which they comment on a target proposition expressed by the accompanying text, as opposed to making an independent contribution to discourse. Focusing on positively valenced and negatively valenced emoji (which we gloss as happy and unhappy, respectively), we argue that the emoji comment on how the target proposition bears on a contextually provided discourse value endorsed by the author. Discourse values embody what an author desires, aspires to, wishes for, or hopes for.

As the study emphasized, facial emoji are distinct types of markers of selfhood, allowing interlocutors to either bridge a social distance with others or else extend it (as the case may be). It comes as no surprise to find that the semiotics of the face as an emotive conveyor of selfhood is intrinsic to the core emoji lexicon. Needless to say, there is significant culturally based variation as to how facial emoji relay emotivity; but at a primary level of expression, there is little doubt as to what emotion they are referencing. It is at the connotative level of meaning that these are interpreted via cultural templates.

When Is It Appropriate and Inappropriate?

Emoji can be appropriate or inappropriate depending on the context and situation in which digital messages are created and received. The data suggests that there is a lack of consensus among healthcare professions with regard to this issue, perhaps reflecting the fact that emoji use is register-less, which might feel anomalous in clinician–patient interactions. All participants agreed that emoji are appropriate for social uses among peers or with any interlocutor with whom they are on a familiar (informal) basis; however, when it comes to professional communicative situations, a difference of opinion emerged. A portion of the participants clearly viewed emoji use in such situations as unprofessional; others instead viewed such use as consistent with digital communications generally, and thus as not impugning the traditional need for maintaining a professional distance with patients via a formal register.

This issue has been found to crystallize across the professional landscape, with social distinctions between workers and leaders, marked by language register, breaking down, as the style of communication on social media is seeping increasingly into all forms of interaction. Interestingly, our study found that "leaders" emerge spontaneously within group formations, with these individuals literally taking the lead in what language, style, or register is appropriate. This finding is also consistent with more general findings that apply to different workplaces, where social stratifications are aligning themselves to new realities created, paradoxically, by the forms of register-less communications that characterize social media discourses. The reluctance to use emoji by some of the practitioners reflects the long-standing belief that individuals need to hold back feelings in professional settings, which would be revealed implicitly via emoji use. This act of self-monitoring informs individuals when it is appropriate to speak up or remain silent, or when to use emoji or not in a communicative situation.

Current research on emotional intelligence in professional communicative contexts suggests that being able to share feelings at relevant moments with coworkers makes the workplace more congenial (for example, Stough et al. 2011). As workplaces have become more diverse and inclusive, organizations have started to realize the value of embracing individual differences and allowing employees to maintain their subjectivity in such settings. This implies that register variables may be obstacles to positive social relationships. So, if one chooses not to use emoji so as to maintain a professional persona for the sake of psychological safety, this same stance today may be interpreted as undermining social cohesion, which might be needed for achieving emotional harmony.

The ambiguity with regard to emoji use in professional settings that emerged from the study is, clearly, characteristic of interactions in workplaces generally. In a relevant study, Amit and colleagues (2022) found that those who used picture-based communications were perceived as less powerful professionally, because they shifted attention away from work-related content to the subjective element in communication. The researchers summarize their findings as follows:

> This research shows people are perceived as less powerful when they use pictures versus words. This effect was found across picture types (company logos, emojis, and photographs) and use contexts (clothing prints, written messages, and Zoom profiles). Mediation analysis and a mediation-by-moderation design show this happens because picture-use signals a greater desire for social proximity (versus distance) than word-use, and a desire for social proximity is associated with lower power. Finally, we find that people strategically use words (pictures) when aiming to signal more (less) power. We refute alternative explanations including differences in the content of pictures and words, the medium's perceived appropriateness, the context's formality, and the target's age and gender. Our research shows pictures and words are not interchangeable means of representation. Rather, they signal distinct social values with reputational consequences.

The data collected from the Palaganas study, however, suggests that the subjective element is actually a conduit for putting coworker relations on a solid grounding. The reactions to the senders of text messages with emoji as to their reasons for using emoji showed that emoji use was appropriate and useful in generating collegiality among peers. Reactions to emoji use were especially favorable when the message recounted some aspect of a person's background or autobiography. In other words, when participants wanted to communicate vulnerability or some other emotive state, they were more likely to use emoji and their colleagues were more likely to react to the messages with emoji themselves.

Why Are Emoji Used (Individually Stated Reasons for Use)?

The opinions stated by the participants with regard to emoji use indicated three primary motivations: (1) the emoji best captured how they were feeling, making it visible to interlocutors concretely (emotivity), (2) they allowed for a sense of engagement with the other interlocutor (phatic communion), and (3) they were effective in shaping the views of one's interlocutors (conativity).

This suggests, overall, that emoji tap into an unconscious need for social bonding, even in professional or educational situations. However, the range of emoji that can achieve this function is highly limited, with selective facial emoji constituting the most used signs in this regard (as mentioned). It may be the sense of inappropriateness that individuals who are not involved in any relationship outside of a professional one may feel, as studies have consistently found (for example, Miller et al. 2016). In a workplace environment, it is unclear when the right or wrong time presents itself to use an emoji – as confirmed by our study. The problem is that emoji can mean many things connotatively and, thus, can often be interpreted in the wrong way, leading to miscommunication. Our interview with Dr. He provided some insights in this area. The gist of his approach is that medical emoji are grounded in a range of meanings that makes them less vulnerable to the usual misinterpretations, given that they are selected specifically to convey medical information in a context-specific way. As such, they enhance medical meaning in an effective way, attenuating the sense of apprehension for miscommunication that would otherwise be intensified, shifting the semiotic lens on empathy. It is no surprise to find that the nurses were most inclined to use emoji, given the centrality of the caring aspect of the nursing profession.

Conclusions

There were a number of interesting findings, along with some limitations, to the Palaganas pilot study. Above all else, it showed that multiple approaches are required to explore emoji uses and literacy, along with multiple sources of data, so as to come to a better understanding of the reasons, motivations, and perceptions pertaining to emoji use in the healthcare professions. There were a number of limitations, needless to say, some of which were related to the nature of the emoji code itself. Emoji types, meanings, and uses change from year to year, so the data collected in 2018 was not isomorphic semiotically and discursively to the data collected in 2022. To maintain a larger sample size, we did not stratify our data per year. This implies that our findings may not apply to future forms of emoji literacy. But, then, this is true of all communicative systems, which are subject to historical forces, no matter if they are verbal, visual, or multimedia-based.

The overall conclusion that can be drawn from the study is that emoji use is perceived, in the end, as effective by healthcare professionals, albeit with some skepticism. The data showed that women in the 30–60 age range, nurses, North Americans, and Australians were more likely to use emoji in professional communication situations. The check mark, thumbs up, laughing face, and heart emoji were the most used, corresponding to patterns in general emoji usage. The other general findings can be summarized as follows:

(1) Emoji use was associated with subjectivity, especially in the recounting of autobiographical events or episodes. This is indirect evidence that a central semiotic function of emoji is episodic annotation (Chapter 7).

(2) The desire for psychological shelter emerged as an antecedent for emoji use.
(3) The participants did not agree as a single group on whether or not emoji are appropriate or inappropriate in health professions due to the critical need in these professions to have clear rules for communications in the area of patient care, avoiding any potential miscommunications.
(4) Emoji are largely used to support others or to convey a sense of empathy.
(5) The study pointed to the likelihood that more and more clinicians will be increasingly open to engaging in emoji communications, not because it is trendy, but because it is relevant and potentially highly effective in the medical world.

Ronald Langacker (1987, 1990, 1999) has argued that the parts of speech invariably evoke unconscious image schemas during discourse. Nouns, for instance, encode the image schema of a region, verbs of some movement in a specific way. It can be argued that emoji evoke image schemas directly, by suggesting nouns or verbs in their visual configurations. This feature of emoji use was found to occur across all the data collected. The participants understood that emoji present content concretely, not in any grammatically defined way. This was consistent with the work of Dr. Cohn, one of the interviewees. In a 2019 study, Cohn came to the following relevant conclusion, on the basis of two experiments he conducted with two other researchers (Cohn et al. 2019):

> Emoji have become a prominent part of interactive digital communication. Here, we ask the questions: does a grammatical system govern the way people use emoji; and how do emoji interact with the grammar of written text? We conducted two experiments that asked participants to have a digital conversation with each other using only emoji (Experiment 1) or to substitute at least one emoji for a word in the sentences (Experiment 2). First, we found that the emoji-only utterances of participants remained at simplistic levels of patterning, primarily appearing as one-unit utterances (as formulaic expressions or responsive emotions) or as linear sequencing (for example, repeating the same emoji or providing an unordered list of semantically related emoji). Emoji playing grammatical roles (i.e., "parts-of-speech") were minimal, and showed little consistency in "word order." Second, emoji were substituted more for nouns and adjectives than verbs, while also typically conveying nonredundant information to the sentences. These findings suggest that, while emoji may follow tendencies in their interactions with grammatical structure in multimodal text-emoji productions, they lack grammatical structure on their own.

Overall, as mentioned and to be discussed further, and as Cohn's own findings suggest, emoji do not possess the kind of grammar of verbal language. As claimed here they have an episodic structure, whereby they are distributed in a message in terms of visual events or states of mind that are interconnected in visual and not grammatical ways (discussed further in Chapter 7).

Epilogue

One general finding that stands out from the Palaganas study is that emoji literacy is starting to be increasingly accepted by the healthcare profession, despite some resistance to it as a professionally inappropriate form of communication. This is consistent with similar findings to be discussed in the next chapter – namely, that the actual interactions based on emoji literacy determine and shape (over time) perceptions of both the messages and the professional senders. Given the empathic nature of a clinician–patient interaction, it would appear that the emoji used are constrained to positive emotivity, and given their episodic structure, they relay relevant episodes of meaning and understanding that are not unlike picture books. As Hand and colleagues (2022) found, in line with the Palaganas findings, message content and emoji type used correspond. The researchers found that: "sentence valence and emoji type interact, influencing message emotionality and clarity, and perceived sender warmth and state." They also found that "emoji typically amplified emotional perceptions of messages and senders."

In another interesting and relevant study, Assadi and colleagues (2020) developed eighty-one medical emoji for a course in which text-based counseling was taught. They achieved a high degree of consensus among the participants as to the usefulness of the emoji, in both inter-provider communications and physician–patient interactions, confirming what Dr. He told us – namely, that emoji are useful devices for both patients and doctors to communicate clearly, effectively, and still maintain the inviolability of doctor–patient relations. As Dr. He also noted, emoji would be particularly effective in interactions with young children, people with disabilities, and patients who speak other languages. Evolving sets of medical emoji, such as the eighty-one already noted, will allow such interactions to be concrete and more precise as well.

Emoji choices are clearly not random when inserted into discourse frames. They are "pieces of meaning" that can either stand alone or else be used to annotate some textual content. As visual episodes in the flow of meaning, they allow users to envisage abstract concepts as implicating each other through a specific image-schematic frame of reference (the emoji itself). Rather than thoughts, evoked by words, emoji evoke perceptions and feelings, which remain vague until an existing "space" in the verbal utterance opens up, wherein appropriate annotations give shape to the underlying thoughts. This implies that user intent becomes prominent in the sense that it imbues the form–content relations that unfold in a message.

The spread of digital communications in healthcare practices provides an empirical framework for studying how emoji discourses can be constrained and shaped to fulfill the needs and functions of professional communications.

Interactive platforms, such as the one used by the Palaganas study, are particularly well suited for both clinicians and patients to transmit visual information that relates to symptoms, pain levels, and other aspects of relevance to diagnosis. In a relevant study of button terminals featuring emoji stationed around hospital emergency departments, Agarwal et al. (2020) found that the emoji were effective in monitoring doctor and patient sentiments in real time. Traditionally, surveys are mailed or sent out electronically to assess patient experiences in emergency room situations, but response rates have been low and have not provided significant information in the past. The study shed light on efficient, rapid ways of identifying trends and providing high-level information on how patients and providers feel in an emergency room situation. The terminals were similar to those used to gauge visitor satisfaction in sports arenas and at airports. Each terminal had four buttons, ranging from very positive (green, with a smiley happy face) to very negative (red, with a smiley frowning face). They were located in three different locations in an urban emergency department to record the sentiments of three specific groups – doctors, nurses, and patients – set up near physician workstations, nurse workstations, and patient exit locations. Nearly 14,000 sentiments were recorded across the three terminals. The nurses' station terminal recorded the most sentiments (53 percent) but, across all three terminals, an average of 108 sentiments were recorded per day.

In sum, studies such as the one reported in this chapter are starting to show that emoji literacy is becoming intrinsic not only to specific pedagogical situations (Chapter 2) but also as an asset to render previously arcane forms of professional communications between clinicians and patients much more amicable and meaningful to the patients. While the project still documented some resistance to emoji use, overall it showed that healthcare professions realize, at the very least, that emoji allow for an effective expression of sentiments, evoking positive emotive reactions – an important psychological factor in treating diseases. The study has also special implications for healthcare education and education more generally (Chapters 5 and 6). Frictionless communication is key in helping to drive quality healthcare, and so, as Dr. He told us, it behooves practitioners to explore ways in which doctors can expand it. In the end, emoji-based interactions have made doctors rethink how they engage with patients and among themselves.

5 Emoji across the Healthcare Landscape

Prologue

In our interview with Dr. Shuhan He (Chapter 4), it was emphasized that investigating the effectiveness and appropriateness of emoji in healthcare-based digital interactions can no longer be put aside by clinicians as mere faddishness. This was one of the key findings, in fact, that has emerged from the research project discussed in the previous chapter, which showed, if nothing else, that emoji use can easily be adopted by health practitioners for various reasons to enhance their interactions with others. The goal of this chapter is to examine emoji use across the healthcare landscape and determine what implications related to emoji theories more generally can be gleaned from such usage and how emoji use can be applied to training healthcare professionals. We will deal with the more general implications for emoji literacy within education more broadly in the next chapter.

In an opinion piece with content similar to the ideas discussed in our interview with Dr. He, Dr. Robert Martinez (2022), a practicing ear, nose, and throat physician, became intrigued by the implications of using emoji in healthcare situations and in public health communications after at first maintaining that "Emojis have no place in medicine," a statement that is consistent with one of our findings (Chapter 4) – namely that some physicians interpret the use of a register-less visual code, based on a popular style of communicating digitally that might seem superficial, cartoonish, and trendy (sometimes called a "pop Esperanto"), as inappropriate for the profession they exercise. But this does not imply that the emoji code is free from perceptions involving social hierarchies; it too is shaped by social power plays, as became obvious with the crystallization of a leader-versus-cheerleader relationship involved in emoji use from the Palaganas study (Chapter 4). As Wiese and Labrenz (2021) also found by analyzing German WhatsApp® messages, emoji use often marks subjective and intersubjective discourse-based meanings, involving social-psychological dominance relations, thus entailing the implicit operation of register, albeit in a different way from its deployment in verbal speech. But, by and large, the same kinds of register functions of verbal speech are either attenuated by the presence of emoji in a message or else eliminated. What Dr. Martinez was alluding to is that a formal level of speech is appropriate in physician–patient interactions – a level that, he at first believed, would render such informal emoji communications anomalous at best and ludicrous at worst.

Martinez brings up his own residency, when he was advised repeatedly to never put anything extraneous or humorous in writing and just to provide facts, free of opinions, and to maintain a social distance from patients via formal language. As he began reading about research on emoji usage in healthcare, he started changing his mind – an outcome that also aligns with the results of the Palaganas study, as skeptical practitioners in the study started gradually seeing the effectiveness of emoji use through interactions with others in the course in which they were enrolled. Martinez sees this type of change in attitude toward the use of emoji as a consequence of the spread of the telehealth interactions that occurred during the COVID-19 pandemic, when clinicians had to learn quickly how to master new forms of communication with their patients on the computer screen, as they witnessed, as Martinez puts it, "patients who were scared and fighting for their lives, isolated from friends and loved ones."

Conducting his own research in this area, Martinez found that emoji add a "human touch" to communicative situations that would otherwise be felt as intense, stressful, and even sterile, thus allowing physicians to convey their concern implicitly (and thus safely), without impugning the seriousness of the clinical communication, while economizing on messaging time and rendering interactions more fluid and interconnected. Martinez's overall conclusion from his investigations forms the theme of this chapter: "Overall the research suggests that emojis [can be] used as a vector for politeness and positive intent in communication among care teams" (Martinez 2022). The question that will guide this chapter is, in fact: Can emoji be used to enhance understanding and break down interpersonal barriers in healthcare situations? The answer appears to be that emoji are, indeed, better able to convey serious information that would otherwise be lost if a patient speaks a different language, cannot quite grasp the complexities of medical terminology, or unconsciously shuts off the impact of negative information because of the threat to their health that it poses.

There is little doubt that changes in technology entail changes in communication style and communicative competencies. At the present time, social media will continue to play a crucial role in public health communication campaigns and in clinical medicine more generally. A simple emoji may provide a critical reminder to take medication (💊), to maintain a healthy diet (🍅 🥕 🫑 🍖 🍆 🥛 🍞), to get vaccinated (💉), and so on, which avoids moralistic tones that can be attached to such advice or counseling. The choice of an emoji in such messages are also interesting in itself, since it involves creativity: What emoji best expresses what I need to communicate? How can I locate it in a message in such a way that it is more effective? With what words can I associate it? Emoji use clearly involves putting together a textual canvas that reflects the ingenuity of each interlocutor via a bimodal system of communicating – verbal and visual – activating a sense of aesthetics that is imprinted in the visuality features of emoji.

The question of politeness raised by Martinez is a key one. In actual fact, there are now implicit rules of "emoji etiquette," which are largely *sui generis*, varying according to situation and context, which makes them unstable and not easily generalizable. Unlike the rules of politeness that are characteristic of face-to-face verbal interactions, which involve words and expressions that are based on register differentiations, the primary etiquette criteria in emoji use involve when to use them and with whom. In digital messages exchanged between those who are on familiar terms, the type and number of emoji used will come down to one's own stylistic preferences and the nature of the relationship between the interlocutors. Even the lack of emoji in such texts communicates a certain type of meaning – as, for example, that something has changed in the relationship or else that the message is a serious one. So, our claim that emoji-based communications are register-less does not imply that they do not involve politeness or etiquette. There are always ways to show deference even via images, albeit in an implicit way. As Yokoi and Jordan (2022) have aptly observed with regard to emoji etiquette:

> Anecdotal evidence, as well as conversations we've had as part of our ongoing research into effective leadership in the digital age, is pointing to the growing use of emojis in the virtual workplace as an alternative to physical cues. They can help clarify meaning behind digital communications, as well as the type and strength of emotions being expressed. But they can also be an intergenerational and cultural minefield. For example, Gen Z's are reportedly offended by their colleagues' use of the smiley face emoji, which they see as patronizing. And cultural and geographical differences can mean that one person's friendly gesture is another's offense.

As psychologist Monica Riordan (2017) found in a relevant study, politeness patterns in emoji use are conveyed via the type of emoji selected for a specific audience – spouse, coworkers, friends, and so on. The different social role we play with each one requires that we relate differently; and it seems that emoji use conveys the relations differentially. A simple example of what it entails to break the politeness protocol in this case would be the use of a poop emoji by a practitioner with a patient, which would hardly be appropriate and rather be perceived as impolite. As Riordan emphasizes, the politeness factor of emoji is negotiated between the interlocutors according to the nature of their relationship – so a clinician would use an emoji differently with a spouse than with a patient, because of the fact that the relationship between them is different and this entails the negotiation of a specific communication style. Emoji etiquette thus helps build and deepen relationships around shared meanings, often becoming "a private language" all its own.

Emoji in Healthcare Communications

Martinez (2022) also issues a caution after analyzing the results of his own survey, since using emoji in the medical world has become an ever-evolving phenomenon that harbors risks, including legal ones:

> In medicine, anything in writing – emoji or not – is part of a legal record. Just as words can sometimes be understood in different ways by different people, that holds true for emojis. I may think the "thumbs up" emoji is the same as answering "yes" to a colleague's question, but what if she doesn't interpret it that way and, as a result, doesn't take an important clinical action? As a doctor, my brain goes there immediately.

The legal issue has parallels in jurisprudence and court cases – an aspect that was hardly anticipated by the creators of emoji, who introduced them as supposed universally accessible and understandable communicative tools to foster benign interactions across the globe, regardless of the backgrounds of the interlocutors. Emoji were viewed, in effect, as positive-sentiment signs designed to engender congenial communication. But, as it has turned out, emoji use, as any kind of language, can be distorted by human cleverness and mendacity. For this reason, Martinez suggests, special attention by the medical profession must be paid to this visual form of communication, even as it serves many benign interactive functions. As Kirley and McMahon (2018: 46) have noted, emoji are being used increasingly as part of deception, characterizing the core of the dilemma that this poses as follows:

> How are we to interpret a message sent by an adult that prima facie appears to contain a threat of violence but is accompanied by a winking face 😉 or a tongue-poking out icon 😛 or 😝? And what are we to make of the man who admitted sending a hostile text message but claimed that the inclusion of an emoticon would lead a reader to understand that "he was merely deeply unhappy rather than sadistically bloodthirsty for revenge"? Clearly, a key issue is the role of positive emoji in either negating or amplifying (in a paradoxical manner) an apparent threat. This moves away from the usual focus on the affective meaning and impact of emoji and instead directs attention to what linguists term illocutionary force: the sender's intention in selecting and using emoji in a particular communication.

This problem of lying and deception has always existed, needless to say. But what limits this possibility in the use of emoji is, as Kirley and McMahon point out, intent – it is unlikely that a clinician would want to use an emoji deceptively in communications with a patient or with other practitioners. The healthcare context itself is an inhibitor of such usage. Of course, lying has been used for the emotional benefit of the patient, although this is becoming rarer and rarer. Emoji misinterpretation is also attenuated in the medical context, since emoji use undergoes semantic and discursive refinement in this area – that is, the emoji are placed in messages to convey a specific meaning and would be interpreted as such, not as harboring ambiguities of various kinds.

So, as Dr. Martinez remarks, despite such potential communicative problems, hospitals, practitioners, and public health agencies can no longer ignore the changes in communications that have taken place since the advent of the Internet, including the use of emoji to shape interactions emotively, especially since, as mentioned, in this area a more honest use of emoji is likely, given the typical content of a message (which involves communicating medical notions and conditions). Even if some patients will deploy emoji for some self-serving reason, and even if practitioners might be misinterpreted, emoji communication tends to be more aboveboard in the medical world; and as in all cases of miscommunications, the problems will be ironed out through actual usage (as the Palaganas research project suggested).

As Meyers and Colturi (2022) emphasize, emoji use in the medical field does indeed appear to achieve "honesty, clarity, confidentiality, comfort, and, when needed, humor, and encouragement," thus enhancing clinician–patient interactions. On the basis of a Doximity poll (an online networking service for medical professionals), the two researchers found that 56 percent of 3,800 clinicians voted yes to the question, "Should clinicians use emoji in a professional setting?" However, a substantial number of clinicians expressed concern that emoji may seem unprofessional or confuse some patients. Moreover, as one clinician observed: "Positive emoji are OK, but negative emoji found in your chart during discovery for some complaint or lawsuit may cost dearly." About 19 percent of clinicians who voted in the poll said that they would use emoji with patients to express gratitude 🙏, empathy 😊, and kudos 👍. Still, many clinicians remain apprehensive about the use of emoji in medicine (34 percent of poll voters). As expected, it was found that the younger clinicians were significantly more likely to advocate for emoji in healthcare than older ones.

When text messaging first became popular and widespread in healthcare settings, practitioners acquired the necessary messaging literacy on their own, along with virtually everyone else, because there was no concrete set of rules, or a special grammar, to compose text messages. So, they set up their own guardrails for using text messaging. Eventually, it became a typical form of interaction among colleagues, and with those patients with whom there was an established dynamic based on familiarity. Text messaging led to a shedding of many of the social-hierarchical connotations that clinical communications tended to encode in the past (Alexander et al. 2021). With the advent of emoji, the same kind of hesitancy has emerged, as Dr. Martinez pointed out, confirmed by both the Palaganas study (Chapter 4) and the Doximity poll mentioned earlier. However, there are concrete expectations, as Martinez suggests.

Like text messaging, emoji use is moving toward broad acceptance, with similar guardrails for such use in medicine being set up.

So, even though emoji communication entails a quasi-register-less speech modality, it has shown itself to be adaptive to the social status of the speakers, their ages, their intent or goal, and so on. As Yang and Liu (2021: 150) aptly observe:

> Another important and probably more general interactive and pragmatic function of emojis is their power in promoting informality and accessibility. In digital communication emojis are usually associated with informality and a casual tone, and they are often assumed to be used more frequently among peers, friends, and relatives. On Weibo, emojis are not only used by ordinary users but have also been incorporated into news briefs and short reports that are publicized by officially acknowledged accounts/users. Once emojis are embedded, the over-all tone of the message becomes less formal and sometimes more approachable, especially with serious genres such as news brief.

A study by Loftinejad et al. (2020) found that emoji use in physician–patient and clinical messaging achieved informality in tone and, as a result, was able to better capture the patient's attention much more than the usual, formalistic, written health messages, such as those imploring people to take hygienic and prophylactic measures in specific public situations. This emotive capacity of emoji became saliently obvious during the COVID-19 pandemic, when emoji use in public health and telehealth communications became common. Due to the immediacy created by COVID, many non-Unicode emoji pictographs were enlisted as visual literacy tools. Table 5.1 presents some such hypothetical emoji used during the pandemic, which show that medical emoji communicate meaning in a compressed and largely unambiguous way.

Table 5.1 *Public health emoji*

Emoji	Implied meaning	Emoji	Implied meaning
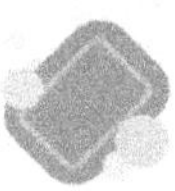	Use soap	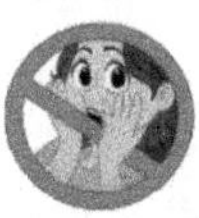	Do not touch your face
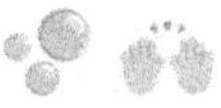	Wash your hands	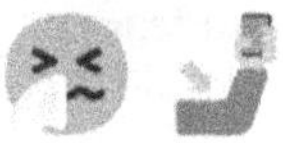	Sneeze into your elbow
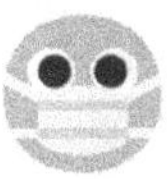	Wear a mask when among people	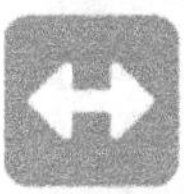	Maintain a distance in public situations
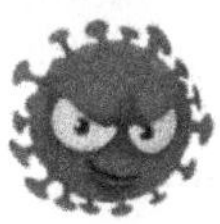	Beware the coronavirus		Warning to take the pandemic seriously

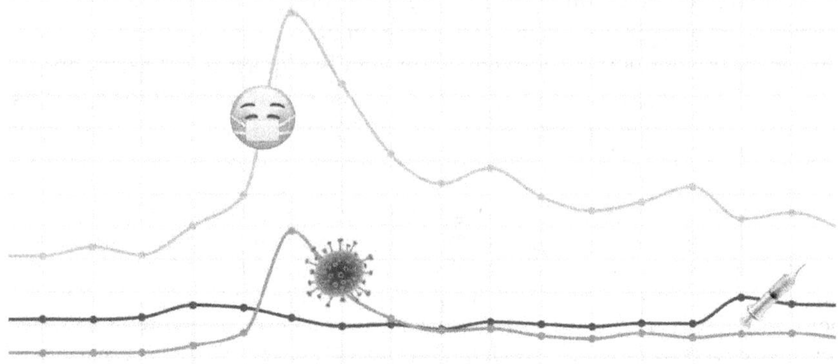

Figure 5.1 Emoji-based graph (from Emojipedia)

Studies have even shown that the use of emoji can make people lean more toward healthier choices in lifestyle and adopting more hygienic behavior, achieving this in a more efficient and less time-consuming way than laborious speeches or written manifestos. Interestingly, the Emojipedia site even published graphs using emoji to show how the pandemic evolved over time, such as the one in Figure 5.1 (from https://blog.emojipedia.org/one-year-on-bored-of-the-pandemic/), which shows Emojipedia's analysis of 976.7 million tweets dated between 2019 and 2021, and how the content of the messages correlated with the spread of the virus, mask-wearing, and vaccinations; as can be seen, the chart is much more effective than a typical scientific one with scientific and mathematical symbols.

Emojipedia's survey of medical emoji showed that, by the end of that year, the novelty of the microbe emoji and the face with mask emoji had waned on Twitter, with a small spike in the syringe emoji . So, as the survey researchers indicated, at the beginning of the pandemic, and during its height, the use of specific medical and public health emoji referencing the coronavirus became intrinsic to communications across the world. Other emoji in the relevant tweets were either highly popular ones, used ironically or reflectively (for example, the face with tears emoji, the rolling on the floor with laughter emoji, the loudly crying face emoji, the warning emoji ⚠, the face screaming in fear emoji, among others). This brings out several things that are pertinent to the present purposes: (1) emoji are now intrinsic as episodic–imagistic–annotative devices, (2) their use during the pandemic was likely a coping mechanism, given that the inbuilt humor in some emoji was likely therapeutic in itself, and (3) emoji had clearly become part of an overall global discourse that had penetrated the professional medical sphere as well. Interestingly, emoji were also utilized by those who were opposed to public health measures during the pandemic, for various contrastive reasons (ideological, subjective, and so on), making their way into politically based debates. The pandemic thus made it obvious that emoji can be used in contrastive ways, again according to intent. That said, the overall effect of the pandemic was to bring about a kind of mini-revolution in the areas of public health and medicine, introducing all kinds of health-related emoji, such as those mentioned earlier. Subsequently, Unicode and Emojipedia have made available all kinds of emoji referring to body parts, such as hands, tongue, eyes, head, teeth, and muscles.

In a pertinent study, Lin and Luo (2023) found that emoji use may actually help shape preventive and self-protective behaviors. With a sample of 210 participants, the researchers found that, compared with nonuse of emoji, the incorporation of emoji in medical communications resulted in generating in patients the awareness of the need to adopt stronger preventive behavioral actions. When emoji were added to health information released by a nonofficial organization, the message outperformed messages from an official agency in persuading people to adopt preventive behaviors.

The foregoing discussion points to the need for imparting emoji literacy to healthcare professionals as part of their general education – as the Palaganas study also suggested. This is especially true in the mental healthcare area, where emoji have been shown to be particularly effective in helping patients cope with their symptoms and mental issues, especially since even the act of starting a conversation on mental health can feel extremely difficult. Emoji are able not only to attenuate the difficulty, but also to destigmatize the discussion – that is, they help remove the negative associations with mental illness. In a relevant study (Van Dam et al. 2019), the researchers aimed to determine if technology-enabled youth therapy, with emoji capabilities, could in fact help clinicians better understand and predict the risks of behavioral health issues for adolescents with mental health problems. Over three months, the participants reported on how they were feeling using one of the icons available in G-Moji, an app developed specifically for this purpose. The results showed that emoji use concretely helped pinpoint positive and negative feelings, suggesting that emoji-based communications in this area have the potential for enhancing both treatment and assessment outcomes.

Clinical Aspects

In a literature review of fMRI studies in psychotherapy, Singh and Hussain (2020) came to the overall conclusion that emoji used in practitioner–patient communications supported our own view that emoji may be used as a healthcare literacy tool to promote well-being (Chapter 3). This finding is not an exceptional one; it appears to surface in many kinds of research projects, even those outside the clinical domain. Among various uses, emoji may be good gauges for assessing well-being. Using a simple questionnaire based on emoji facial expressions with young children, Allen et al. (2017) found that emoji signs could be used profitably to assess well-being levels in young children. The researchers found, initially, that parents and teachers consistently scored children's happiness levels higher than the children scored their own. The team then decided to consult the children directly, using a questionnaire with emoji faces representing moods and states of mind and asking the children to rate how they felt in various situations by selecting the appropriate emoji, such as on the way to school, in the classroom, in the playground, and so on. From this, they found out what the children's moods really were, in contrast with those attributed to them by adults. The emoji tool had opened up a channel of meaningful conversation with the children, allowing them to talk openly (without any sense of fear or menace) about their feelings, giving them a voice, particularly around key decisions that affected them. A corroborative follow-up study was conducted by Riad et al. (2021), which also found that self-report tools are better suited to evaluate children's well-being.

In the clinical area, studies have come forth to corroborate the utility of emoji tools for assessing levels of well-being. In a 2022 study, conducted by Davies, McKenna, Denner, Bayley, and Morgan, an emoji-based questionnaire was used to measure well-being and mental health in a range of settings and services outside of conventional mental healthcare settings. Two groups of participants were selected: (1) one that completed an online questionnaire containing emoji-based categories and (2) a group that completed instead a traditional-type questionnaire. The questionnaires were designed to assess mental health, resilience, community connection, and well-being. A third group completed a paper-and-pencil version of the emoji questionnaire (in offline situations). The researchers found that the emoji-based tools provided a compact and consistent measure of mood and current experience across the participants, while those who completed the traditional questionnaire showed a higher variability. It is likely the length of the usual formal measuring tools that makes them impractical for use, especially where time is short or when assessing individuals who do not possess the required literacy levels. In order to be inclusive and accurately capture self-reports in a meaningful way, studies such as this one suggest that emoji cues may provide the best way to assay well-being levels.

The relation between emoji usage and well-being is, clearly, a key area for healthcare research and attendant practices (Chapter 3). In a significant study by the Mayo Clinic (Dangor 2017), researchers found that using emoji instead of the traditional emotional scales and charts was much more helpful, and accurate, in assessing cancer patients' physical, emotional, and overall sense of their quality of life. The study employed Apple's ResearchKit, which provides objective, continuous activity data that can be used to assess cancer patient-reported outcomes. ResearchKit allows practitioners to build apps that allow for the routine assessment of well-being. Cancer patients face medical and financial consequences that can negatively impact their well-being and quality of life. Since these play an important role in predicting survival and determining the best treatment options, identifying them is critical. The study showed, in addition, that wearable technology data correlated positively with traditional, validated patient-reported outcome measures. The research involved 115 patients with lymphoma and multiple myeloma at the Mayo Clinic with expected life spans of less than five years. Each patient owned an iPhone, and all patients were provided with an Apple Watch at the start of the project. Researchers collected baseline data, including questions regarding physical functions, levels of fatigue, ability to sleep, perception of social roles, and views on quality of life. The researchers also developed emoji scales to measure the latter characteristic. During the first week of the study, the patients wore the Apple Watch for an average of 9.3 hours per day, were required to take 3,760 mean steps per day, and exercised 8.3 minutes per day, allowing for 224.9 sedentary minutes. The researchers observed significant associations between standard patient-reported outcome measures and the collected activity data. They also found that the patients' emoji responses correlated positively with the outcomes.

In another relevant study, Callender and colleagues (2022) found that conventional survey methods to determine states of mental health do not capture emotional fluctuations in any useful way. So, they tested the feasibility and validity of gathering data on Therapeutic Radiography student mental well-being during clinical placement via emoji. The participants were asked to provide anonymous daily emoji responses via WhatsApp to a dedicated mobile phone. Additional weekly prompts were employed to seek out textual responses on matters of well-being. The fifteen participants used 108 different emoji, which were triangulated with the weekly textual responses. As it turned out, the happy smiley face emoji was used most frequently. Szeto et al. (2022) conducted a general review of the relevant literature in this area, assessing the possible healthcare applications of emoji as tools for assessing and even promoting well-being. From their extensive literature search, they were able to identify how, why, and when emoji were employed in communications concerning general healthcare, pediatric healthcare, public health, and dermatology. Among the themes that stand out, the researchers found the following: (1) emoji tend to improve communication within pediatric healthcare; (2) they are effective in capturing mood and mental health patterns; (3) they provide a basis for developing interventions to improve patient medication adherence; (4) they complement novel (new media) channels of public health surveillance; and (5) they bolster dermatology-specific applications.

As the studies indicate overall, the medical repurposing of emoji presents many advantages over the usual methods, especially given their register-less tone and inclusivity. As Liu (2023) found, patients are more likely to answer questions about their well-being more honestly via emoji communications because of these inbuilt features, finding again that the happy smiley emoji appears to be the one most often selected to acknowledge either a state of happiness or a desire to reach this state.

Diseases occur in the body, but reactions to them can be influenced by the signs used in clinician–patient interactions, which can even influence the course of a disease, since they have the capacity to generate brain chemicals that are beneficial to stemming the course of a disease, as more general research in this area has suggested (Rankin 2013). It might well be that emoji generate a kind of placebo effect; that is, it may not be farfetched to hypothesize that with the boost from the positive sentiments associated with emoji, the healing process is enhanced. Evidence that this may be the case comes from a 2023 study of clinical depression patients by Kandola et al. (2023), which used self-management digital apps with emoji to determine if they aided patients who self-identified as having depression, scoring 5 or more on the Patient Health Questionnaire-8 (used to assess mental states). The participants were randomly assigned to receive the app for eight weeks or a limited attention-placebo control version of the app. The results showed that use of the app reduced symptoms of depression at eight weeks significantly more than the symptoms experienced by the control group.

The overall conclusion that can be tentatively drawn from the studies is that emoji might affect patients positively. Constant stress has an adverse effect, whereas positive feelings and relaxation return the body to its normal state and may thus boost the immune system. Emoji are not medical cures in themselves, needless to say; they are simple pictures that affect patients positively, much like humor. They may also counteract the so-called nocebo effect, defined as a detrimental effect on health produced by psychological or psychosomatic factors such as negative expectations of treatment or prognosis. So, there is some reason to believe that emoji can play a healing role in an overall (holistic) approach to therapy, since they appear to be mood enhancers.

A comprehensive survey in this area was the one conducted by PerfectServe in 2022, a provider of cloud-based clinical collaboration (www.perfectserve.com/the-rise-of-emoji-in-healthcare-communication/). The study revealed that emoji have a specific positive function in medical environments compared to the way they are used by the general public. Specifically, the survey found the following differences:

- The thumbs up emoji was the one most frequently used by clinicians across the board to signal acknowledgment.

- Among the top ten emoji used by clinicians versus the top ten used in the general population, only the face with tears of joy appeared on both lists. This emphasizes the uniqueness of professional clinical communications, which are intended to be generally more positive in tone, indicating perhaps that clinicians are developing their own communication protocols with emoji.
- Internal medicine was the top specialty for emoji usage. Second place on the list was orthopedics, followed by physical medicine and rehabilitation.
- Practitioners used emoji more than other care team members, including nurses and case managers.
- Among the medically themed emoji, the face with medical mask showed up most frequently, followed by the microbe emoji.
- The research confirmed that emoji are used to convey politeness and positive intent without sacrificing professionalism.

Clinician–Patient Interactions

As healthcare communications and interactions have become almost exclusively digital, clinicians are grappling with how to comport themselves professionally, while embracing the positive aspects that the new technology offers, as the research discussed previously strongly suggests. This has had an impact on clinician–patient communications (Chapter 3). In an overview of relevant studies, Sharma (2023) found, in fact, that emoji-based communications between doctors and their patients are increasingly common, mainly because they provide clarity in difficult situations, at the same time that the tone of positivity built into the emoji enhances patient understanding. As Dr. Shuhan He told us in our interview with him (Chapter 4), a substantial addition to the lexicon in the area of medical emoji is thus crucial in this area, even though this might cause some confusion at first, given the context-based and often subjective nature of emoji interpretation. As he understood, the degree of exactness between the real experience of symptoms and the emoji is not an isomorphic one. Nonetheless, as per any communicative system, the meanings of the medical emoji are contextualized within specific semantic-episodic boundaries – communicating medical conditions.

One area that is especially relevant is when emoji can be used as suggestive conceptual gap fillers when a language, or a patient, does not have a term for, or understanding of, some disease. Consider rickets – a childhood disease caused by vitamin D deficiency, characterized by the softening and distortion of the bones, ending typically in bow legs. The disease may be present in the body without someone realizing that this is so, remaining unrecognized and untreated. The patient may see the distortions as part of some genetic inheritance, rather an actual physiological disease caused by lack of vitamin D. When someone without knowledge of rickets is diagnosed with rickets, the practitioner might have to inform them that the condition is not a legacy of genetic inheritance but the result of a dietary deficiency. This might actually take some convincing, as has been shown by public health studies of rickets (Bivins 2007). So, the first stage in the treatment process is a fundamentally semiotic-discursive one – namely, to convince sufferers that they do indeed have a disease, so that a meaningful medical-therapeutic engagement can be ascertained. For instance, to define the disease via visuality, emoji based on illustrations could be used, since these show the effects of rickets in a powerful visual way.

Very few people are diagnosed with rickets anymore. If they are, they are not usually in countries where they would be texting with the doctor anyway. So, the following discussion may be somewhat constrained, but it is used nonetheless to indicate how emoji could (hypothetically) be employed in conveying the meaning of any disease. Successful diagnosis involves, in some part, a strategic, probing dialogue with patients that will allow clinicians to contextualize the symptoms, psychologically and culturally. This "diagnostic interaction" is critical in the early stages of a disease, because it is useful to determine the actual symptoms as reported by the patient, and thus provide a means for diagnosing a malady in concrete terms. The use of emoji in digital interactions might also establish a crucial emotive and phatic link between clinician and patient, which may support the smooth flow of the diagnostic interaction. A study by medical practitioners O'Reilly-Shah et al. (2018) found that emoji use did indeed enhance teleconsultation interactions, not only between physicians and patients but also within the medical community itself, such as interactions between doctors and doctors, doctors and nurses, and nurses and nurses.

As an example of how emoji can be allocated in a digital dialogue, for the purpose of making something concretely understandable, consider a hypothetical online dialogue between a doctor and a patient who may be suffering from rickets, with the patient having no idea what rickets is. The emoji used in the diagnostic interaction are placed strategically so that the overall meaning of rickets can be stitched together conceptually by the patient.

PHYSICIAN: For how long have you had these symptoms ?
PATIENT: Since I was a child.
PHYSICIAN: Do you know why?
PATIENT: No.
PHYSICIAN: Do you consume dairy ?
PATIENT: Almost never; I am lactose intolerant to a degree.
PHYSICIAN: What about or liver?
PATIENT: Occasionally, eggs.
PHYSICIAN: Do you know what D is?
PATIENT: I learned about it in school.

PHYSICIAN:	Would you agree that you have been getting very little vitamin D because of your diet?
PATIENT:	I guess.
PHYSICIAN:	Lack of vitamin D is the likely cause of your symptoms. In medicine your condition is called rickets . It is a serious disease.
PATIENT:	Oh, what should I do?
PHYSICIAN:	Now that you know, we can start to take action, OK?
PATIENT:	OK.

A primary goal of the hypothetical dialogue is to make the patient aware of the relevant background (cultural, lifestyle) factors that supported the doctor's diagnosis, via visualization, rather than just words, which often bear judgmental connotations. The dialogue, albeit hypothetical, is not unlike the kind that is used by practitioners in similar real-life situations. Note as well that the textual part retains a higher register of communication that is blended with the register-less one associated with the emoji – constituting a stylistic blend that is common in such interactions. Nonetheless, even though the choice of most of the emoji is neutral in sentiment, there are touches of imagistic humor in the emoji, not unlike the kinds of verbal witticisms that a doctor might use in a face-to-face conversation. Diagnostic interactions such as this have actually been found to promote cooperative speech (as discussed earlier). Returning to our hypothetical example, once the diagnosis has been explained to the patient, the same positivity of tone can be achieved through emoji that relate to therapy:

PHYSICIAN:	As you now understand, you have a condition that needs your attention. Don't you agree?
PATIENT:	I do, thank you.
PHYSICIAN:	One thing you can do right away is to alter your diet. You can eat more such as salmon. You should also get more , since it is a major source of D.
PATIENT:	Yes, I will try.
PHYSICIAN:	Great, but be sure about this. As you know, I am always here to help you out .
PATIENT:	Well, I might have some difficulties adjusting.
PHYSICIAN:	Of course. But I know you will try, right ?
PATIENT:	Yes.

One might think that the allocation of the emoji in such dialogues is purely descriptive or decorative, or even artificial, simply reinforcing the verbal part or perhaps confusing in itself; but this is not correct. If one removes the emoji and just leaves the textual part, it becomes obvious that the dialogue will be lacking something. This is because the emoji in the dialogue annotate the content, providing visual information associated with it that adds to the overall holistic effect of the message, as well as establishing a congenial tone.

Moreover, they invite the patient to construct a visual, nontechnical portrait of medical information. The hybrid dialogue can thus be said to effectively convey technical information in an agreeable and highly comprehensible way, with the emoji distributed cohesively in the text to allow for the mental image-schematic composition of the disease and the required therapy. Wood and Ruder (2016) see this use of emoji as a key feature, indicating that their annotative function becomes powerfully suggestive when it is distributed through the selected emoji as a guide to the meaning.

As Nicole Najda (2016) has shown, this kind of annotative-distributive style is critical in therapeutic contexts. Observing conversations among aphasic individuals in institutional settings, she came to understand the importance of ensuring a positive tone in the flow of conversation as a concrete therapeutic strategy. Aphasia is becoming a major problem because of age-related conditions, such as the incidence of strokes in elderly individuals, resulting in difficulty in speech. Her research found that communication among aphasic partners in institutional settings involved a variety of strategies to promote the flow of conversation that made sense to elderly interlocutors, including the positivity that the dialogues enfolded. She concluded that therapists enhance their success rates when they speak positively to aphasic speakers.

A schematic list of the annotative features of emoji in medical dialogues and public health communications is the following:

- *Humor nuances*. They can make technical jargon understandable in line with current modes of online communication (such as some types of videos on YouTube, including TED ones that involve medicine), adding humor nuances to make the disease emotionally manageable. This communicative pattern became prominent during the COVID-19 pandemic. Coronavirus emoji were used by various public health sites to (paradoxically) convey the seriousness of the disease. Below are three such emoji, which are designed to convey the importance of being aware of the danger of the coronavirus, portrayed with a sinister look, and to grasp how the virus instilled fear and panic:

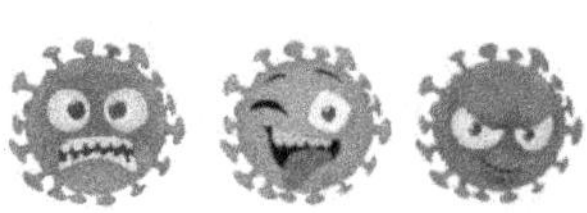

- *Polysemy*. Different emoji for the same disease can take on different nuances of meaning (polysemy) according to their form and their location in a message. The smiley emoji used earlier in our hypothetical dialogue, , allowed the doctor to convey concern and availability; needless to say, it might have ironic meaning if used to critique a patient for not following a prescribed regimen of medication or therapy. But this is rare, as the relevant literature has indicated.

- *Code decipherment.* The word *rickets* refers to a specific type of malady; it is literally a key to unlocking the disease code. The emoji used by our hypothetical doctor (, , etc.) are keys to that code and its dietary basis. The term *code* as used here is in line with the practice in semiotics (Saussure 1916), defined as a specific system of signs that bear specific kinds of meanings.
- *Contextualization.* Emoji such as those used in our hypothetical dialogue can be seen to contextualize something abstract, such as a disease, allocating it within the patient's social and psychological life. The food emoji contextualize the disease in a dietary way, while medical therapies, such as the use of vitamin D, are contextualized in different ways, such as the need for getting more sun indicated by the sun emoji ( ).
- *Clustering.* When used in clusters, annotative emoji provide emphasis with regard to a medical condition. For example, the dietary aspects of rickets could be summarized with a cluster such as the following:

Annotative emoji have been shown to be especially effective in the treatment of mental diseases, as some of the studies discussed in this chapter (and in previous ones) have shown. This may be a result of the iconic force of the emoji to represent changes in mood, personality, personal habits, or social relations that many mental illnesses bring about. As Dr. He told us, they are especially effective in fleshing out misconceptions about illnesses. In a relevant study, Dr. He and a team of researchers (He et al. 2022) used emoji scales to annotate pain thresholds (see also Brown 2022): The team found that such emoji preloaded onto electronic devices provided a highly accessible, user-friendly, no-cost method for collecting and storing clinically relevant patient information, particularly from young children and individuals with culturally and linguistically diverse backgrounds. In other words, the scale turned out to be an accurate, open-source, and economical alternative to the usual analog pain scales. In the mental health area, the relevant studies have also shown that people exposed to emoji-using communications developed more favorable views of mentally challenged individuals, thus potentially attenuating the social stigma that patients may feel about their disease. The same destigmatization can be arguably achieved in all areas of clinical medicine, since annotative emoji provide a visual means for understanding, coping with, and presumably developing the strength needed to overcome a stigma.

The foregoing discussion implies that emoji could be tailored annotatively and episodically to complement the doctor's communicative repertoire in conveying some disease or malady to patients. Following are our own illustrative examples, which are meant to show how different emoji provide snapshots of diseases in nonthreatening and destigmatizing ways:

(1) *Malaria*: The symptoms include an intermittent and remittent fever caused by a protozoan parasite that invades the red blood cells. The parasite is usually transmitted by mosquitoes. The word *malaria* was coined by physicians in the eighteenth century, from Italian *mal aria*, which means "bad air" thus alluding metaphorically to the original belief that the disease was a product of an unwholesome atmosphere caused by the exhalations of marshes. Relevant emoji that could be used in combination for this disease are the following (which associate it with mosquitoes, including the mosquito act of blood sucking):

  🦟 🩸

(2) *Cancer*: The disease is caused by an uncontrolled division of abnormal cells in a part of the body, often resulting in a malignant growth or tumor. The word *cancer* is derived from Latin, meaning "crab or creeping ulcer," which is a translation of Greek *karkinos*. The name is a metaphor that came into use when physicians became aware that the swollen veins around tumors resembled the limbs of a crab. There is currently no breast cancer emoji. However, since the commonly accepted symbol for breast cancer is a pink ribbon, groups such as EmojiRequest.com have petitioned Unicode for such a depiction to be created and adopted into the lexicon. The emoji would look like 🎗 but pink. Until its adoption, a theoretical representation of breast cancer may perhaps be simulated as:

  🎗️ ♀️

(3) *Paralysis*: This term denotes loss of the ability to move and sometimes feel anything in part or most of the body. It results typically from an illness, poison, or injury. The word was coined from Latin via Greek *paraluesthai* meaning "to be disabled at the side," which is a metaphorical blend: *para* "beside" + *luein* "loosen." Emoji signs in this area include the following, which show the results of living with some paralysis-based disability, requiring the use of a wheelchair:

  🧑‍🦼 🧑‍🦽 🧑‍🦼

(4) *Diabetes*: This term describes a metabolic disorder that occurs when the body does not produce enough insulin, leading to an excess of sugar in the blood that causes excessive thirst and the production of large quantities of

urine. It derives from the Greek metaphor *diabainen* ("siphon"), in reference to the excessive discharge of urine as if in a siphon. Also involved in diabetes is hypoglycemia, or low blood sugar, caused by medications used to treat diabetes such as insulin, which produces an array of symptoms. Facial emoji used portray these symptoms have been developed, for example, by the Diabetes Research Institute.

(5) *Eczema*: This refers to a condition in which patches of skin become rough and inflamed, with blisters that can cause itching and bleeding. The term comes from Greek *ekzein* "to boil over, break out." The following theoretical emoji shows where eczema might occur on the body, warning a patient visually against scratching the affected area (in this case, the arm):

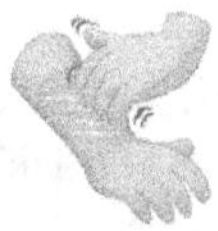

(6) *Rubella*: This refers to a contagious viral disease, with symptoms similar to measles. It is a color metaphor, from Latin *rubellus* (plural *rubella*), meaning "reddish." It occurs mainly in childhood, so the theoretical emoji below might be constrained to communicating the disease and its symptoms to children; they also portray how sick one might feel from experiencing the disease and the need to stay in bed:

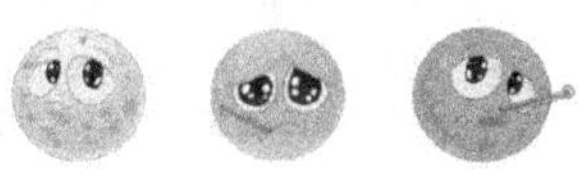

(7) *Influenza*: This term denotes a contagious viral infection of the respiratory passages causing fever, aching, and catarrh. It is an Italian word meaning, literally, "influence," from medieval Latin *influentia*. It was applied for the first time to an influenza epidemic that began in Italy in 1743. Symptom emoji for influenza might include the following:

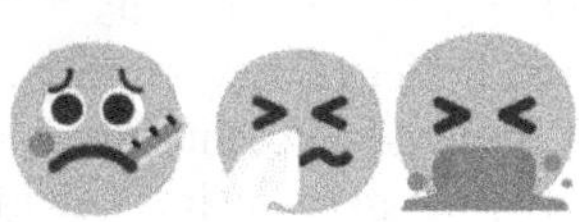

(8) *Asthma*: The term refers to a respiratory condition marked by spasms in the lungs, causing difficulty in breathing. It derives from Greek *azein* "to breathe hard," which describes the main symptom itself. Combined relevant annotative emoji in this case might include the following:

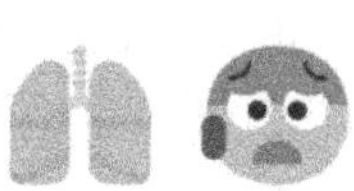

A first impression might be that these are cartoonish images that have no other effect than to lower the level of a medical dialogue to that of a comic book. However, because emoji are now part of a generic visual literacy, which is embedded in the conveyance of humorous nuances in interactions (virtually by default), the use of such emoji is not out of sync with general communicative practices in the culture of the Internet. So, it is unlikely that they will be perceived as unbefitting of how a doctor should communicate, as the PerfectServe survey found (see earlier in this chapter). In some medical contexts it may well be out of character, but in most clinician–patient interactions, which are grounded in familiarity, the use of emoji is simply an up-to-date manner of communicating that is highly understandable and amiable, without compromising perceptions of expertise and seriousness. Abundant evidence exists highlighting the positive physical and psychological health benefits of humor (for example, Farifteh et al. 2014; Savage et al. 2017). In effect, emoji come with an inbuilt laughter "eye track" (to use a paraphrase of "soundtrack").

The overall intent of using emoji in clinician–patient interactions, or in public health communications more generally, no matter how cartoonish they might seem, is to provide a visual and congenial portraiture of diseases that can help the patient grasp the seriousness of the condition in non-fearful ways, which itself will facilitate medical diagnosis and treatment (as discussed). It also conveys an unconscious sense of caring that might not be achievable otherwise. Emoji use in such situations involves a visualization strategy, that is, the use of emoji to create easy-to-communicate and easy-to-understand content for a broader, non–medically trained audience, to help them visually explore and discover, understand, interpret, and gain insights into otherwise complex ideas. They are also usable to convey a concise version of known information in a clear and engaging manner. As Thomas and Cook (2005: 30) aptly observe, visual representations "take advantage of the human eye's broad bandwidth pathway into the mind to allow users to see, explore, and understand large amounts of information at once … conveying abstract information in intuitive ways." Moreover, the patient does not have to learn any sophisticated ideas or methods to be able to interpret the emoji annotations.

As mentioned several times, however, there are caveats with respect to the use of emoji in healthcare situations. One of these is the enthusiasm that some doctors show, which might be misinterpreted by the patients in a negative way. Also, there are doctors who do not use emoji, and this could constitute a needless unconscious competition among doctors for gaining patient attention. Moreover, not all patients are emoji-literate or inclined to see emoji as a viable or socially appropriate way of communicating in medical situations. Another caveat relates to the culturally, gender-, and age-based differences in emoji use, perception, and meaning connotations. This could easily cause confusion in patients unnecessarily. Also, the degree of exactness between the experiences of a patient and the use of emoji is unclear, requiring further research. Finally, as Dr. Martinez warned (cited at the start of this chapter), there may arise legal issues related to emoji-based communications, yet another area that requires further investigation. All that said, the evidence in favor of using emoji in healthcare-based communications is rather substantive.

As discussed in this book, emoji do not conform to the same register dichotomies of verbal speech, but they do enfold etiquette and, thus, politeness modalities that are interweaved into the overall sense of friendly respect that they build into a medical message. As the PerfectServe platform concluded following its survey (see earlier in this chapter): "This suggests that emoji can be a tool for building camaraderie and lightening the emotional load in an environment that is frequently fast-paced and stressful."

Implications for Healthcare Education

One of the salient implications emanating from studies on emoji use in healthcare and studies of the use of emoji in literacy training (Chapter 2) is that emoji are now part of a general form of communication that blends verbality and visuality in synthetic (bimodal) ways. So, emoji can, and should, play a greater role in education. Since this chapter has dealt with emoji in the healthcare world, we conclude it with considerations of why and how emoji can be used in training healthcare professionals, following up on the pedagogical implications of the results of the study in Chapter 4. We will look at the more general issue of emoji use in other areas of education in the next chapter.

As studies and surveys have shown, the use of emoji in medical situations is now spreading. So, among the first things that will have to be imparted to healthcare students is an understanding of the emoji code and its variable interpretive modalities. This would include presenting, discussing, illustrating, and providing appropriate materials on the following issues:

- the sign-based differential modalities of emoji (iconicity, indexicality, symbolism) and how these allow for the expression of various types of meanings;
- the connotative (polysemic) aspects of emoji, including the variation in form and content associated with the emoji platform;
- the culturally based interpretive diversification of the same emoji, and the specific range of emoji types preferred by different cultures;
- the differences in expression encoded by scripts that are based on verbality and those on visuality; also included in this area is the use of multimedia resources to reinforce a message and when and if they are appropriate;
- a sentiment analysis associated with the different facial emoji;
- a pragmatic assessment of the semiotic and discourse functions of emoji (emotive, phatic, conative, etc.);

- a discourse analysis of how some emoji project nonverbal cues in face-to-face interactions onto the screen (including gesture, microexpressions, etc.);
- a discussion of the illustrative–annotative functions of emoji in medical texts;
- a presentation of the metaphorical qualities of some emoji and how they are interpreted differentially according to context, situation, and in response to variables such as age and gender;
- a discussion of how the location of emoji in messages is an episodic function that allows the overall meaning of the text to be interlinked via the distribution of emoji within the message;
- a discussion of the potential legal and interpretive dangers of emoji use;
- comparisons between medical usages of emoji and those of the general population, including how emoji dialects have emerged based on geography and the emergence of Internet slang;
- a discussion of destigmatization and socially sensitive justice issues that are connected with emoji use, given its register-less qualities, without comprising politeness and etiquette.

An issue that needs particular discussion in the medical classroom is the perception of emoji as part of a pop culture trend that does not belong in medicine. Traditionally, medical students are told that they must abide by the highest standards of professional conduct, leaving little room for humor. This is not surprising because of the nature of humor, which is problematic in certain contexts, bearing perhaps unwanted connotations. But emoji seem to step around this, given that they are capsules (no pun intended) of humor without verbal commentary – a form of suggestive humor that can sidestep the usual interpretive setbacks of verbal jokes. And given the communicative culture in which patients (and doctors) now live, humorous touches in therapy and consultations may be seen as essential – the lack of such touches may come across as a lack of empathy. Regardless of where clinicians stand on emoji in medicine, their use requires carefulness and understanding. It is akin to teaching medical students how to convey compassion.

The continuing studies course described in Chapter 4 showed how training in emoji use emerges spontaneously through concrete interactions among peers. It also showed that there is no need to learn emoji as a language with its differential vocabulary and grammar from, say, English. It is an understandable image-schematic mode of relating meaning that varies according to user and context, constituting a kind of "visual code-in-use" that is intuitive rather than formalistic.

One salient feature of emoji use in an educational setting, as the literacy study described in Chapter 2 indicates, is that they tend to grab the immediate attention of students. A study by Kim and colleagues (2022) showed, in fact, that medical students were more attentive in online courses when emoji were involved in pedagogical and inter-group communications, finding in particular that the use of emoji in professor–student communications was a motivating factor in this regard. The study hypothesized that a "professor's use of emojis in a welcome letter could result in the enhancement of psychological relationships with student recipients, such as students' perceived authenticity and intimacy with the professor, leading to increased intrinsic learning motivation and sustained attention in the professor's online class." The sample consisted of 297 students in public universities in the United States. Data were collected via a scenario-based survey approach. The result showed that emoji-based communications led students to perceive the professor as "authentic and friendly, making students more intrinsically motivated and more inclined to pay attention in the professor's online class."

By the very nature of emoji, and as our own research has suggested, a central feature that the use of emoji in education entails is that it presents communication in an edusemiotic intuitive way, even if the instructor is not aware that it involves semiotics; that is, the emoji themselves put on display the various types, levels, and modalities of signs. The end result is the development of an unconscious competence in what has been called semioliteracy here (Chapter 2), or the control of different signs and sign systems in a holistic, integrative fashion, with the ability to navigate verbal and nonverbal meanings through it – a competence that is highly relevant in the Internet age. The semioliterate aspects of using emoji systematically include the following:

(1) Students become intuitively aware that signs and sign systems share properties based on meaning intent. While emoji are visual signs, they reinforce the verbal signs, which then correlates with holistic (presentational) forms of meaning-making, in contrast to discrete ones as pertaining to the monolithic use of words.
(2) Another key principle that might be acquired intuitively is that differences in the manifestations of sign properties are due to the histories and traditions of particular cultures and societies. Since emoji emerged at the same time throughout the world, one would assume that they have universal or common properties of signification. This has not turned out to be the case, as discussed. Nevertheless, a core lexicon (typically made up of facial emoji) is much more inclined to produce semantic similarities in usage and interpretation, no matter the cultural backgrounds of the interlocutors.
(3) Signs and sign systems entail culture-specific classifications of the world. This is essentially a corollary of the previous principle.
(4) They influence the way people think, behave, and act. As the studies discussed in this book have shown, emoji usage influences perception of emotive and phatic meaning, reshaping the way people communicate such functions.

(5) The facial emoji signs are assumed to naturally represent something, whereas the truth of the matter is that there must be consensus as to the interpretive range that these capture.

Pedagogically, it may well be useful to include emoji as devices for imparting knowledge by making it enjoyable to the students, who are themselves users of the emoji outside of the classroom. That is, using emoji to present medical information as annotative devices might produce a learning transfer effect. Psychologist Edward Tolman (1932) used the term "cognitive map" to describe how the extraction of ideas from experience guides their subsequent use in related tasks. He called this kind of behavior "latent," since it occurs without any reinforcement of the behavior that was learned previously. Tolman's idea is useful for understanding how emoji might have a "cognitive mapping" effect, allowing learners to find their way through the verbal information contained in complex areas of medicine via a bimodal flow, as it has been called here (Chapter 2), given that they are based on visual processing that constitutes a basis for cognitive map building.

Emoji can be included generally under the rubric of visualization training, which requires that students weave together their own background knowledge, experiences, and creativity to develop image schemas of what medical information entails. Like a geographical map, this might allow them to retain the conceptual location (so to speak) of some notion in the mind more lastingly than by memorization of concepts presented in verbal script.

Epilogue

We started this chapter by citing a medical practitioner who was initially skeptical about emoji use in his own practice, and thus resistant to the kind of seemingly nonserious interactions that it implied, but who eventually realized that emoji use was simply part of how people communicate in the Internet age, facilitating many aspects of clinician–patient interactions, including those that involved serious content, given that emoji shaped the conversation in an amiable fashion, without destroying the actual content, but rather annotating it in its own way. A similar reaction was noted in some of the participants in the Palaganas study discussed in the previous chapter.

Emoji communication is spreading throughout the healthcare world. However, as in any professional arena, it will require a discussion about appropriate protocols in emoji uses so that professionalism can be ensured. The studies discussed in this chapter point to a broadening awareness in healthcare interactions and education that languages and communicative practices are in constant flux, and thus, for clinicians to be able to communicate in a more relevant and meaningful way with patients, emoji literacy cannot be marginalized but must instead be used and studied as to any relevant changes that might occur. As McLuhan emphasized throughout his career, even before the advent of the Internet, as the technologies of mass communications change, so too does groupthink. The main semiotic problem with emoji is that of the interpretant (as discussed several times). What do emoji communicate, and does intent match their use? Are emoji actual speech forms, and does that mean they are protected? As emoji crop up in all sorts of situations, medical and legal, they raise such questions about professional communication. That said, there is no doubt that they are integral tokens of digital speech.

The study of emoji in a healthcare context involves discussions in areas such as medical ethics, medical anthropology, and others. This will lead, in our view, to important research on the connection between disease (the body), patient perceptions of disease (the mind), medically sensitive communicative styles and codes (dialogue), and the contexts in which the disease emerges (culture). As J. F. Barnum (1993: 939) has insightfully remarked:

> Diagnosis will succeed only to the extent that we respect the principles and caveats of sign interpretation. The sign is both the key to the unknown and the master impersonator. The sign and its meaning are usually not the same; meaning has to be inferred. Because interpretations are made subjectively, they are circumscribed by the experience and bias of the clinician. Moreover, the contexts in which the sign appears shape the meaning of the sign and may change it altogether.

Concepts of health and disease crystallize due to a combination of social, cultural, legal, and scientific factors, not from any strictly clinical analysis of disease. That is to say, cognizance of a particular disease crystallizes by observing not only symptoms but also what it means in a culture. Recall the example of acne (Chapter 3), found commonly in areas of the world in which unhealthy eating habits are common, especially among adolescents. To reiterate, it is characterized by inflamed sebaceous glands in the skin and by red pimples on the face. In urban societies such as the United States, England, Canada, and Australia, acne afflicts a substantive percent of the adolescent population. In the early 1990s, Swedish medical researcher Staffan Lindburg (1994) visited the island of Kitava in the Trobriand Islands group off Papa New Guinea, finding no evidence whatsoever of acne among any of the denizens. Lindburg attributed this to the healthy diet of the Kitava people. The medical and public health implications were apparent to everyone – acne is a skin disease connected with culture – it is not caused by exposure to some bacterium or virus or by some internal degenerative process, but by eating habits. In effect, the diagnosis and treatment of acne cannot occur without taking into account this broader picture. Disease and health are products of the body, mind, and culture influencing one another reciprocally.

The case of acne actually shows what the semioliterate consciousness of a disease might entail – namely, a knowledge of how symptoms might fall on a three-dimensional scale of iconicity, indexicality, and symbolism.

Table 5.2 *The semiotics of acne*

Type	Sign	Examples
icon	The symptoms of acne can be represented by an emoji that stands directly for the actual physical symptoms, such as the presence of pustules on the face.	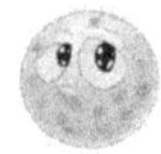
index	At this level acne is mapped against its relation to diet – foods and drinks high in sugar and carbohydrates that tend to get into the blood quickly.	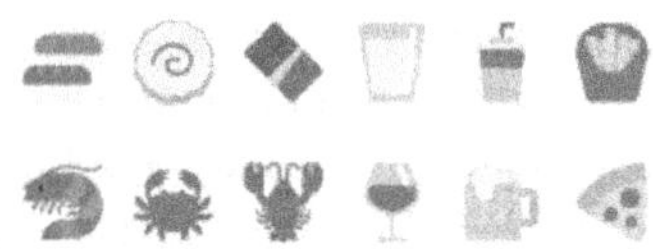
symbol	Acne produces facial furuncles, which might generate negative cultural perceptions. To avoid this, and to treat acne as a dietary-induced condition, low-glycemic foods are prescribed.	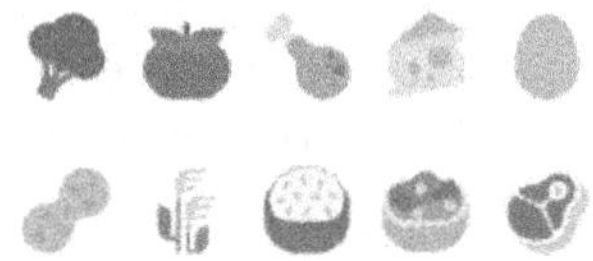

Mapping these against emoji characters might allow young patients to grasp the meaning of acne, medically, and what to do about it (Table 5.2).

As this example shows in microcosm, semioliteracy is at the core of decoding meaning in a holistic (multidimensional way). In an extensive review of the relevant literature, Szeto et al. (2022) found that, in dermatological treatments (such as acne), emoji do indeed play a key role as signs that work psychologically at different levels of comprehension. As such they improved communications within pediatric healthcare, enhancing mood and helping develop interventions that the patients would accept and adhere to. They also found that emoji helped monitor the side effects of dermatological treatments. In similar studies on chronic pruritus, patients of dermatology preferred self-reporting their itch symptoms with a cartoon emoji-based scale called "ItchyQuant" over a purely numerical scale or some other quantitative scale. To wit: medical practitioners and students of medicine should be aware of emoji literacy and its connection to semioliteracy when diagnosing interactively with patients, so as to allow them to navigate the best personalized care for their needs.

6 Emoji in General Education

Prologue

English teacher Martin Sketchley (2022) recounts a pertinent experience of using emoji as teaching-learning devices to support the acquisition of English as a second language by his online learners, most of whom had little or no background familiarity with the language. He exemplifies his approach in various interesting and pertinent ways. For example, he uses one and two apple emoji (with written words) to illustrate the difference between singular and plural. He adds the happy-faced smiley emoji for the verb "like" and the sad one for "not like," thus connecting the semantics of the verb "like" to its expected microexpressions. In effect, this little illustrative pedagogical presentation encapsulates how emoji can be incorporated easily and directly into pedagogical practices.

On a psychological level, this type of pedagogy makes no assumptions as to what the learner should (or should not) know already about the object of study. As discussed (Chapter 2), emoji use involves inclusivity by the very nature of the signs, which are not marked for social level and thus will not elicit judgmental critiques, as would the choice of words that are tagged unconsciously for such things as class and intellect. Given that emoji are used in parallel ways by virtually everyone who has a computer or mobile device to communicate, such counterproductive distinctions are eliminated from classroom learning. In effect, the emoji tend to ensure that the learners in Sketchley's online course will not feel excluded intellectually, but will rather engage as participants in the learning process via the familiarity that they undoubtedly have with emoji usage. Such pedagogy is clearly both inclusive as to student intellectual backgrounds and effective as a means to activate semiotic mechanisms that are unconscious, such as the relation between form and meaning (such as the plural structure and the notion of referential number). The emoji devices are, in effect, mediators from one system (emoji) to another (the English language).

For beginning levels of learning, emoji provide a simple, yet cognitively powerful, pedagogical method for imparting new knowledge. One of the main implications that the research discussed in previous chapters, such as the study by Petcoff on the use of emoji as a basis for imparting literacy to developmental students (Chapter 2) and the use of emoji to facilitate communications in the healthcare field (Chapter 4), is that emoji do indeed have concrete, meaningful roles to play in areas such as education and the training of healthcare professionals. Further investigating and discussing these roles is the objective of the present chapter. Our underlying premise is that emoji not only are highly understandable images, aiding learning but can also create a positive environment, making teaching and interaction congenial and open to all learners, no matter their backgrounds or learning capacities, since emoji give them an equal voice (Fane et al. 2018). As we saw and argued in previous chapters, emoji allow for a destigmatized approach to disadvantaged learners who might not be able to adequately speak for themselves. They are a psychological conduit that can easily open up the lines of interaction to virtually everyone.

A subtext of this chapter is that the way we read and write messages may indicate a shift in how our consciousness and relation to the world are evolving, away from the linear mode of processing information, characteristic of the print age, toward a more holistic mode, characteristic of artistic expression. If so, then the way we perceive how learning is supposed to take place in formal settings is evolving as well along the same lines. The new literacies that have emerged as a result of new technologies, which have migrated to all areas of society, can be classified under the broad rubric of semioliteracy, as it has been called here. This involves knowledge and control of the diverse verbal and nonverbal semiotic systems that define the amalgam of literacies that have crystallized today. Some critics (for example, Helprin 2009) see these negatively, claiming that they are producing an addictive "dumbing-down" effect on how people process information, rendering them much less pensive and reflective as they were, presumably, in the print age. Others have responded that they reflect nothing more than an effective new way to create messages based on the technologies (Crystal 2011). Emoji writing does not imply that people have lost the desire to read and reflect upon the world. On the contrary, it can become a bridge to that world open to all kinds of learners. Moreover, emoji may contribute to counteracting learning challenges, such as dyslexia, as relevant studies now indicate. For example, Lesniak and Grzybowski (2021) found that emoji (and emoticons) helped dyslexic learners improve their ability to read and understand texts.

In sum, emoji literacy has a broad range of implications for education. Emoji broaden communicative competence to include a system of semiotic portrayal that involves the ability to blend verbality and visuality, emphasizing the interrelations between different cognitive states, not their separation. This has concrete implications for education in different types of subject matter, as the Sketchley example previously brought out in microcosm.

Emoji in the Classroom

The relation between emoji, well-being in the classroom, and enhanced learning outcomes was studied concretely by Fane et al. (2018), corroborating, overall, that emoji convey positive emotivity, despite the (relatively rare) potential for misinterpretations, which, as discussed here, can be tamed by familiarity of usage within a given context (a hospital, a clinician's interaction with patients, an educational setting, etc.). The Fane study used emoji with seventy-eight preschool children to investigate how they understood and experienced well-being, discovering that they opened up learning to novel input effectively on their own without the need for any special type of intervention.

Using core facial emoji, the researchers found that these presented children with optimal opportunities to assert easily how they experienced well-being. The study's findings point to the ability of emoji to engage and involve all voices in any situation – they are nondiscriminatory signs by their very nature. As the researchers claimed, the written word is privileged and more under the control of adults than children, allowing them to speak for the children. As a result, the children's voices are excluded due to their preliterate status. With the advent of multimedia literacies and the growing recognition of the need to include everyone's perspectives in matters such as education, emoji are emerging as a valuable tool in early childhood settings, giving young children a concrete way to communicate and explore their emotions and ideas through the emoji code. Above all else, as the Petcoff study (Chapter 2) showed, they make students feel safe in expressing themselves without fear of reprobation. Also, since emoji are neutral as to social and cultural variables (by and large), they offer opportunities for freely exploring knowledge in the classroom without any perceived constraints as to background. As such, emoji bring a hospitable atmosphere to the classroom, especially in cases where learning is difficult for students for various reasons. Emoji tap into the contemporary fascination with all things digital, creating conditions for learning mechanisms to become activated spontaneously. They also stimulate creativity since stories or explanations can be composed with emoji that allow students to utilize them in imaginative ways to convey their perspectives, bringing these out visually through the emoji signs. Since emoji are not right or wrong, as is for example a misspelled word, they encourage a positive transfer effect to other areas of understanding where they would be perceived as nonjudgmental and could thus help students unconsciously understand and thus better utilize standard language for academic reasons.

From another relevant angle, by including emoji formally in the classroom, as did Sketchley (see beginning of this chapter), the teacher would be speaking the language of the students, which would allow the teacher to transform that language into a medium for connecting with them at different psychological levels. Needless to say, not all young people are motivated to learn in this way; but then, these do not need any particular pedagogical approach to aid them in the learning process. However, even in such cases, emoji-based education can channel everyday literacy practices to make discussions and illustrations in class enjoyable. As the Sketchley example indicates, emoji can be envisaged as a pedagogical metalanguage that can be used to shed (visual) light on concepts and allow students to use them to grasp abstractions. Emoji can also be used profitably to give feedback on digital work. Critical feedback can sometimes come across as harsh, even if not intended to be so, but using emoji has an inbuilt positive emotive effect that can make receiving feedback a little less unpleasant. Research suggests in fact that when providing feedback, emoji soften critiques that may lead to hurt feelings or conflict. Moffitt, Padgett, and Grieve (2021) found that criticism containing even a single smiley face emoji will be perceived more positively than criticism without it. Moreover, if located at relevant spots in the feedback, emoji can draw the student's attention to the area needing further work. As Kharbach (2022) has remarked, effective teaching involves the ability to "capitalize on affective communicative strength to boost students [sic] communication and enhance their socio-emotional learning." The relevant literature suggests, in fact, that emoji-based pedagogy does indeed help meet student social-emotional learning needs (for example, Li et al. 2021) and cultivate social presence – the ability to perceive and include others in a mediated environment (Andel et al. 2020). In effect, as the Petcoff study also found, emoji help build a crucial rapport between teachers and students that arguably activates natural learning processes in itself.

Some teachers may see emoji as unprofessional in the education context, as doctors also do in their own contexts (Chapter 5), but the research literature suggests that their use has no detrimental impact on the level of professionalism or competence that students perceive with regard to their teachers. Despite the enthusiasm of some educators today in adopting emoji for pedagogical reasons, the same array of caveats that apply to emoji use in general would apply to education settings as well. First and foremost is the question of meaning, making it necessary that students and teacher develop a common ground of understanding with regard to what the core lexicon emoji mean. This is essential in preventing any misunderstanding that might arise. The top twenty or so emoji are the usual ones that we ourselves found to surface in our studies, namely the facial emoji (Chapters 2 and 4). However, even in this area, caution is required. The blushing face emoji, for example, is supposed to denote that the sender is embarrassed but could be misinterpreted, since metaphor and other figurative processes could enfold an array of unwanted meanings for the classroom, including affection, attraction, or admiration, which are associated with pink cheeks.

Standing back and examining the emoji-in-education trend that is gaining a foothold in some areas of the world, it can be argued that it reflects the ideas of John Dewey and Marshall McLuhan, which were put forth before the Internet age. Dewey (1902, 1916) argued that education is a social, interactive process, not an individualistic one based on the intelligence levels of students. He believed that students thrive in an environment where they are allowed to experience and take part in their own learning, emphasizing that the classroom was not only a place to gain content knowledge or skill in some discipline but also a locus to learn how to live in the real world by bringing that world into the classroom, including its communicative and symbolic artifacts. McLuhan (1969) went further in emphasizing the need to incorporate into the classroom the communicative patterns that were evolving in the global village via connective technologies. He realized long before the Internet age that such technologies impel us to become more involved with one another, no matter what language we speak or in what culture we were reared. As a result, McLuhan envisioned that technology had made what he called a "classroom without walls" a reality (McLuhan 1960). The isolated classroom with a single teacher instructing and interacting with a small group of students in one specific region of the world belonged to the print age; it is now an anachronism in the global village. Emoji can be said to bring the language of that village into the traditional walled-in classroom, transforming it, ipso facto, into a McLuhanian classroom. Of course, even in the print age, educators and students were able to access and share ideas beyond the classroom. But it involved physically going outside the classroom to interact with others, making it much more laborious and unmotivating to many students.

In a prescient way, McLuhan (1960: 3) saw the radical educational changes that the digital world would bring about long before these came into existence:

> These new developments, under quiet analytic survey, point to a basic strategy of culture for the classroom. When the printed book first appeared, it threatened the oral procedures of teaching and created the classroom as we now know it. Instead of making his own text, his own dictionary, his own grammar, the student started out with these tools. He could study not one but several languages. Today these new media threaten, instead to merely reinforce, the procedures of this traditional classroom. It's customary to answer this threat with denunciations of the unfortunate character and effect of movies and TV, just as the comic book was feared and scorned and rejected from the classroom. Its good and bad features in form and content, when carefully set beside other kinds of art and narrative, could have become a major asset to the teacher.

Education in the digitalized global village, as McLuhan anticipated, is on the threshold of a paradigm shift, because we now live on both sides of the computer screen. This implies that we are subject to the communicative laws of both real and hyperreal space – the space on the other side of the screen, to use a term made famous by the late French philosopher Jean Baudrillard (1983).

As teacher Carrie Foster (2018) remarks, the "art of great communication is making a message relevant to the audience for which it is intended," and this can only happen today if the signs for conveying relevance that are found in hyperreality are incorporated into communication.

Emoji Pedagogy

Teachers have always brought in materials from the world outside the classroom to make the learning process more practical and relevant. Emoji clearly fit into this pattern. It thus comes as no surprise to find that educators and teachers themselves are turning more and more to social media-based pedagogy as a way to make the classroom meaningful and relevant. At the turn of the twentieth century, children engaged with school subjects by listening in class to the teacher, reading textbooks, and practicing what they had learned via exercise manuals or written assignments handed out in class. They had no voice in the matter. Pedagogy was teacher centered and based on prepared materials that were used in a standardized way across school boards. The primary revolution that the Internet age has engendered is that students are now provided with many opportunities to shape the learning process interactively with teachers.

Given this paradigm shift, questions of what emoji pedagogy might entail concretely are now cropping up throughout the educational world. We started this chapter citing the pedagogical perspective of English teacher Martin Sketchley (2022), who proposed an emoji-based pedagogy for teaching English as a second language through an online course. Earlier we looked at his example of how he used emoji to teach nouns and their plural formation. Another example from his article regards connecting English adjectives to feelings and moods by simply using facial emoji displaying different feelings and then asking users to connect these to adjectives such as *exhausted*, *hilarious*, and so on. As in his previous example, the emoji cues are part of a visual instructional metalanguage – that is, they are themselves elements not to be learned but to be used to help students learn something – in this case a subset of adjectives. The "guessed translation" part of his methodology allows the students to transfer what they have learned visually to the actual language. As Sketchley then suggests, there should be brief follow-up discussion sessions for learners, getting them to reflect on the lexicon and grammar that was learned indirectly, as well as the creation of a story based on the lesson, with emoji as gap-filling prompts.

Examples such as the ones described by Sketchley show concretely that emoji pedagogy is easily realizable and limited only by the needs and imagination of the teacher. Another case in point pertains to the work of Holton and Symons (2021), who describe various instances of teaching mathematics via an emoji metalanguage to bolster learning, since they can support understanding of processes such as algebraic representation in primary school, without any prior knowledge of algebra, given that emoji are essentially contemporary ways to carry out the "visual representation of a dynamic object that presents opportunities for construction of mathematical knowledge" (Moyer et al. 2002: 372).

McCaffrey and Matthews (2017) call this type of approach "emoji math," to describe how equations can be solved using emoji in place of traditional symbols, thus bringing the outside world of communications into the classroom as well as using a visual language that is much more easily decipherable than a purely math-symbolic one. One aspect that must be always kept in mind, however, is the kind of emoji used. If, for instance, a pepper emoji is used as an algebraic variable, this might generate unwanted meanings in a classroom of adolescents in particular. It is one of the caveats that we have mentioned throughout this book. That said, it is saliently obvious that this method allows students to look at math in a new way, which is based on signs that emoji math, and emoji pedagogy more generally, can help students unlock abstract ideas more intuitively than, say, with variables such as x, y, and z. McCaffrey and Matthews are aware that this approach, while engaging and accessible, may appear to be faddism and to "dumb down" mathematics. In response, the authors make the following case (McCaffrey and Matthews 2017): "The algebra represented in [the emoji system] is not dumbed down at all. Notice that the puzzle presents a linear system in three variables. First-year algebra students are generally not exposed to three-variable systems." The key principle is that emoji equations provide a useful metalanguage for getting students to transition from emoji math to more formal algebra, rather than starting with abstract symbols, which might leave too many students behind.

There are now a plethora of websites offering examples of emoji math resources that can be applied to any classroom. In effect, emoji pedagogy provides a concrete entry point into abstract notions, whether they are of grammar or algebra. As educator Doiron (2018) comments, the main strength of emoji pedagogy is that it recognizes how students grasp meaning through emoji pictography. Doiron suggests that the selected (or constructed) emoji be contextualized for purpose and meaning, so as to avoid the pitfalls described previously.

Literacy Training

In Chapter 2, we described and discussed a study by Petcoff that indicated concretely how emoji literacy could be used as the basis for imparting academic literacy, involving a group of students who were enrolled in a developmental reading and writing course as compared to students in a regular first-year writing class. To reiterate here, the goal of the study was to evaluate if the incorporation of emoji literacy into the developmental classroom was effective in getting those students up to college readiness levels, mastering writing skills similar to those taught in the paired credit-level course. The study thus has direct implications for using emoji as a viable writing instruction tool more generally – that is, across diverse student populations. In part, the study was motivated by the relative lack of materials for literacy instruction to remedial students, which, Petcoff realized, contributed to making the situation worse for teaching developmental learners. Reading and writing instructors have typically had to craft learning tools that could be used profitably in such cases. The use of emoji in the classroom turned out to be a highly effective way to fill the gap – allowing students to feel involved in the learning process, given their familiarity with emoji. The result of the study indicated that emoji pedagogy in literacy training does indeed help developmental students gain the same levels of academic literacy of their peers in regular classes. As Elizabeth Losh (2015) has remarked, such results should not be surprising, because pedagogical activities that revolve around materials and ideas with which students are already familiar will help them gain better control of new subject matter, and especially the semiotic connection between levels of literacy and their applications in the real world. She also suggests that multimedia-delivered courses, including graphic novels, video games, and the like, allow the teacher to translate their content into reflective discussions of important social themes such as injustice and prejudice.

In a relevant work, Gray and Holmes (2020) looked at the interconnection between code, culture, and practice as a way to analyze emoji literacy as a form of a new rhetorical style. Understanding digital signs such as emoji requires understanding the rhetorical possibilities that these make available through an amalgamation of verbality and visuality. Rhetorical thinking is central in all views of what literacy entails in the domain of persuasive discourse. The ever-expanding lexicon of emoji bears witness, in part, to the need to make emoji rhetorically available discourse signs, which, as Gallagher and Avgoustopoulos (2023) argue, requires the Unicode Consortium to think literally outside its own box, since persuasive signs cannot be inserted into a universalist box of understanding. On the other hand, one can never lose sight of the need to make any universalist-aspiring semiotic code as inclusive as possible. This line of reasoning has clear implications for literacy training in a diverse classroom where assumptions as to student background and knowledge about the nature of rhetorical discourse and its nuances cannot be made. In an in-depth literature review, Barinaga-López et al. (2022) found that inclusivity considerations have rarely been studied per se, although research has been expanding in showing how emoji implicitly (unconsciously) entail inclusivity by their visual nature, as discussed throughout this book.

The discussion of emoji literacy and its role in educational settings for imparting traditional academic literacy leads to a historical consideration of what literacy means and what it entails psychologically and socially. The relation between a language and a society that uses it can be sought in the nature and function of the writing system used for both official and informal communication purposes, along with the value ascribed to writing as a means to gain social status. As mentioned, before the advent of alphabets, people communicated and passed on knowledge through the spoken word. But even in early cultures, tools had been invented for recording and preserving ideas in pictographic form. So instinctive is pictography as a mode of writing that it comes as little surprise to find that it has not disappeared from our own modern world, even though most of written communication in western societies is based on the alphabet. It manifests itself in forms of representation that range from arrows in public places to indicate directions to the use of illustrations in textbooks and even scientific treatises. As discussed in this book, this blending of verbality and visuality is an important one psychologically, since it entails blending various regions of the brain that perform R-Mode and L-Mode functions, so that a holistic mental picture of something emerges with verbal and visual elements.

Writing serves a host of social functions. Without it, modern-day society would be unrecognizable. Books, magazines, online blogs, websites, and all the other forms of communication that are based on writing and that we use on a daily basis for a host of functions, from information-gathering to entertainment, are central to maintaining modern-day social systems. Traditionally, individuals who are literate – essentially those who can read and write – are those who have always wielded authority and influence throughout history. Before the 1400s, the vast majority of people were illiterate. Most had never had an opportunity to learn to read because there were few schools, and books were scarce and often expensive. Although some people at every level of society could read, most literate people belonged to the upper classes. Literacy spread at an uneven rate until the invention of the printing press in the 1400s. Marshall McLuhan (1962) characterized the world that this event engendered as the Gutenberg Galaxy, after the European inventor of the printing press, German printer Johannes Gutenberg. Through books, newspapers, pamphlets, and posters, McLuhan argued, the printed word became, after the fifteenth century, the primary means for the propagation of knowledge and ideas. More importantly, given the fact that books could cross national boundaries, the printing press set in motion the globalization of literacy for spreading ideas, paving the way for the European Renaissance, the Protestant Reformation, and the Enlightenment. With the spread of commerce and industry during the eighteenth and nineteenth centuries, large numbers of people migrated to cities where they were forced to learn how to read instructions and perform other tasks that required literacy. Governments began to favorably value the social roles of educated (literate) citizens, no matter what class they came from; as a result, systems of public schooling expanded. By the late 1800s, basic education had become largely obligatory. More people had the opportunity and motivation to learn to read and write, causing the literacy rate to rise rapidly. Today, literacy is still considered to be the primary means for gaining social mobility, prestige, and economic well-being. But the notion of literacy has diversified considerably, becoming even more associated with technologies beyond print. So, the term is no longer constrained to mean the ability to extract meaning from print and the ability to put meaning into print. It now covers parallel abilities in nonverbal forms of representation, from the purely visual (such as emoji literacy) to the control of highly technical systems (such as coding literacy in the area of computers).

To this day, academic literacy remains a primary form of literacy, involving language at higher levels of grammatical, lexical, and stylistic usage; and it is still gained in school, now alongside other literacies. Gaining such literacy means being able to engage in written (and especially technical and highly reflective) texts of all kinds. In using emoji as a conduit to such literacy, the idea is that it provides learners a metalanguage that will allow them to engage with academic-technical texts in ways that bear communicative meaning to them. We use the term metalanguage in this area in the same sense as discussed earlier in emoji math, that is, as a visual tool that encourages students to translate the emoji forms into verbal (literate) counterparts. In no way does this imply that emoji are not, in themselves, autonomous signs with their own vast array of functions (as discussed throughout). Verbal language is also used metalinguistically all the time in the classroom – language to teach about language, for example. The emoji metalinguistic function can be more productive because it is distinct from the verbal metalanguage (which reverses upon itself in teaching), and thus much more able to allow students to focus on the language as the target of study, not as both target and source. This certainly makes teaching much less confusing. Needless to say, this means that the stock of emoji available for use must be enlarged, or at least refined pedagogically, so that it can cover the required domains of learning.

Of course, emoji themselves are new vehicles for expressing our thoughts, feelings, and reactions. So, they play a dual role in literacy training – as self-contained signs that can even replace verbal writing in total, if the need should arise, and as complementary signs that reinforce meaning but also illustrate learning material in a metalinguistic way. Emoji pedagogy, consequently, eliminates (or at least attenuates) the judgmental sense that writing style assigns the individual to a particular class or group. Emoji are essentially classless, used by individuals across social categories. That is why their use in the classroom injects a sense of inclusivity, as the Petcoff study clearly showed, allowing students who might otherwise feel excluded or marginalized to feel included in the classroom in equal ways. The specific types of speech patterns that reflect social power alignments and ideological relations among groups is thus removed from the classroom. To change institutions and social practices implies changing the discourses used by those who have a stake in them, to paraphrase the late philosopher Michel Foucault (1972).

As Mikhail Bakhtin (1981: 80) has observed in a pertinent way: "Many people who have an excellent command of a language often feel quite helpless in certain spheres of communication because they do not have a practical command of the generic forms used in the given spheres." A native speaker of English who is perfectly fluent in the language might still not be able to write an academic paper according to the proper conventions of that genre. But through the medium of emoji literacy that same speaker might gain insights into how writing and style of expression might interact, much like the emoji math pedagogy (discussed earlier) is able to show the relation between spheres of representation – the abstract and the visual (emoji) – in an easy-to-understand, concrete way. As the relevant studies suggest, the use of emoji as part of literacy training appears to set in motion a transfer effect, whereby through observational mechanisms such as an instinctive or intuitive comparison between the two forms of literacy (emoji and academic), students may be more inclined to apply the skills they have learned via such training to academic writing.

The question of what differentiates emoji literacy from traditional literacy is a relevant one, since it is the flow from the main features of one form to the other that guides the metalinguistic learning process. These can be charted as in Table 6.1.

Emoji literacy is based on the retrieval of visuality, which, as Catherine Moore (2017) has aptly pointed out, has always been a part of how we communicate in symbols. Visual writing has always been a complement to verbal

Table 6.1 *Emoji versus traditional literacy*

Feature	Emoji	Traditional	Metalinguistic function
referentiality	image-based	word-based	the holistic versus discrete nature of emoji versus words may raise awareness of how meaning can be encoded differentially
organization	episodic	syntax	the arrangement of episodes to imply a visual story raises awareness about the nature of order itself as a syntactic phenomenon
semantics	annotative meanings	word and phrase meanings	may raise awareness of how semantic considerations shape the content of a message
stylistic	distributive	conventional	the ways in which emoji are distributed in a message coherently might raise awareness of how literary style is itself a coherent system based on conventions

writing, producing two types of literacy that have been united via the common hybrid code (emoji + words) that is used today. As Marissa King (2016) has aptly pointed out, from a practical standpoint, a key attribute that emoji bring to the classroom is that the students are themselves the "literati" in this case, and their competence in emoji literacy can be exploited advantageously by engaging them to demonstrate and explain the implicit "rules" for using emoji – episodic, semantic, and social – and then discuss what differential rules must be acquired to control traditional verbal literacy. This provides a congenial situation for motivating students to become agents in transferring their digital forms of literacy to the traditional form. As Petcoff found (Chapter 2), teachers do not need to be emoji experts to use them in the classroom, nor do they need to keep up to date with changes in the emoji rules, especially since it is impossible to freeze them at any point in time, given the fluidity of the emoji code. As King (2016) suggests:

> Welcoming emojis into the classroom is one way to use student experience to develop school skills. Rather than detract from learning goals, our students' rich social media lives can contribute to deeper learning. By connecting to skills our students already use online, perhaps we can make school seem even more relevant.

In another relevant work, Sexton and Beegle (2020) provide a set of practical pedagogical ideas and examples of how emoji literacy can be incorporated into the teaching of academic literacy – also portraying the usage as a didactic (metalinguistic) transfer strategy to facilitate the acquisition of academic literacy. By purposefully incorporating emoji into everyday instructional practices, the authors suggest, the teaching process becomes itself enriched.

What all this shows, in a nutshell, is how emoji are always available as pedagogical devices that can be easily adopted and adapted to the classroom to guide specific learning tasks (Crombie 2020). In a sense, emoji are contemporary rebuses, which represent ideas (usually expressed in words) by a picture; several rebuses may be combined to make a phrase or sentence. In Renaissance Italy, rebuses were employed both to communicate with people who did not read and to teach literacy.

To test anecdotally if teachers were using, or would use, emoji in their classrooms for reasons such as those discussed previously, a phone survey was used by one of the authors of this book (Danesi) with five teachers in the city of Toronto at the elementary school level, selected because they did not use emoji in their teaching. The informal conversations revolved around the possibility of using them. From the responses of four – one did not use contemporary technologies at all – the following opinions were collated:

(1) *Idea-sharing.* It was pointed out by all the teachers interviewed that a function of emoji use could be to allow students to share ideas in a

contemporary way. One teacher stated that emoji might also reduce tensions that sometimes arise from the face-to-face mode of interaction, which may be daunting to some students, especially shy ones.

(2) *Congeniality.* Three of the teachers stated that allowing the use of emoji for various in-class communicative tasks was a way to make the classroom a congenial one, thus favoring learning.

(3) *Specific teaching tasks.* When pedagogical proposals such as the ones discussed in this chapter (including emoji math) were described to the teachers, they reacted positively, indicating various ways that they themselves could use emoji to carry out their own teaching tasks.

(4) *Reinforcement.* One teacher saw emoji use as a technique to reinforce learning, given that they could be used annotatively to allow the student to review something learned via the visual channel.

(5) *Multimedia-based approach.* All teachers saw the possibility of using emoji as part of multimedia-based teaching, tapping into the ways in which students today read texts on their screens.

(6) *Supplementary teaching aid.* One teacher saw emoji use as a supplement to teaching, rather than a complement, claiming, rather insightfully, that students might otherwise start to envision the "emoji-immersed" classroom, as she put it, as a means to escape real effortful study.

(7) *Foster interaction.* All interviewees agreed that, if nothing else, emoji had the capacity to foster interaction in the classroom.

(8) *Personalization.* Two teachers believed that emoji would allow students in the class to add their own thoughts at any point in time about content and classroom atmosphere in a nonthreatening way.

(9) *Discussion of issues.* Political, social, and other kinds of issues are typically tagged with hashtags and emoji on social media. Two teachers mentioned that such symbolic forms might have great value in bringing these issues to the classroom without bias.

(10) *Grammar.* One teacher, who taught English, pointed out that emoji could be used easily to impart grammatical ideas, reacting to the example presented to her of using facial emoji to teach adjectives. She also cautioned, however, that some parts of speech cannot be represented by emoji – these include prepositions, conjunctions, and the like.

(11) *Vocabulary.* When presented with research that showed that emoji provided opportunities for building vocabulary and reading skills, all agreed that this was a viable use of emoji. However, one teacher pointed out that there is a caveat – what an emoji means to one person is not the same as what it means to another. However, it was also believed that discussing differences and finding the words that represent them is potentially a way for students to build vocabulary.

(12) *Constructive criticism.* Using emoji in grading and various assessment forms was seen by one teacher as a very useful aspect of emoji, since, as he emphasized, it diminishes the sense of failure, providing instead implicit encouragement.
(13) *Writing stories.* Interspersing emoji as annotative devices in a story assignment was seen as very useful by one teacher. She also pointed out that illustrated stories have been used since time immemorial to help children learn to read and write, and thus that emoji would simply provide a means of updating this technique.
(14) *Summarizing text.* Everyone agreed with the principle that emoji provide understandable ways of breaking down and summarizing texts, via their allocation at various points in the text. One teacher used the example of how an emoji can be used to indicate how a character is feeling or acting at a certain point in the narrative.
(15) *Providing feedback.* As one interviewee pointed out, teachers had been putting smiley and frowning faces on student work for years before the emoji phenomenon. Emoji would thus offer a more current way to do the same thing.

A theme repeated by both teachers who use emoji, and those who might do so, is that they help fulfill students' socio-emotional needs, offering an opportunity for meaningful interaction and understanding in a socially humane environment (Zhou and Landa 2021). Emoji pedagogies also allow teachers to meet the challenging reality of learning in a world that is dominated by ever-changing technologies. This may be short-lived, since technological changes bring about changes in communication patterns and styles. So, the pedagogical principles and ideas that apply to emoji pedagogy can also be seen as providing a foundation on which to prepare for future changes. Much like their use in healthcare communication systems (Chapter 5), the adoption of emoji in classrooms is part of a communicative-learning management system, with emoji use as a point of departure for establishing contact and providing instructional content that is much more easily understandable. As discussed, moreover, although a specific emoji may have various meanings, its interpretation tends to be significantly similar for students within the same discourse community. Given their visual nature, emoji allow students to express personal narratives (episodic function), progress on learning tasks (metalinguistic function), and seek assurance (emotive function).

To obviate the perception of emoji use as potentially random, without students knowing the exact learning purpose for their use or also appearing to be frivolous teaching devices, as one of our interviewees pointed out, they should be utilized systematically and nonexclusively; that is, with other techniques (Zhou and Landa 2021). Overall, emoji pedagogy involves reimagining content and methods of imparting skills in ways the technology presents and diffuses throughout society.

Emoji as Visual Rhetoric

From their inception as emoticons, emoji have served as rhetorical signs broadly. A corollary of the Petcoff study (Chapter 2) has been that emoji are, in many instances, rhetorical projections, via their annotative, emotive, phatic, and episodic functions in particular, allowing interlocutors to visually create a message through depictions of people, places, and objects, constituting a form of inherent visual rhetoric. Among the implications for teaching that this central feature of emoji might have, the following are worth highlighting (Petcoff 2023):

- Emoji can serve as part of a visual system of understanding. As Lebduska (2014) observes: "At the end of the day, emojis are just as much a reflection of their creators as words, with just as much potential to express, explore, kvetch, and ultimately connect us to others. Though in some instances they supplant words entirely, they also open up new vistas of exchange and creativity."
- As Gray and Holmes (2020) assert, emoji can be used to bring out the rhetorical force of a message and, thus, to instill in users the awareness of the power of image schemas to shape ideas and to guide interpretation (conativity).
- Since emoji design varies from one platform to another, this presents an occasion for the teacher and student to examine the intrinsic relation between form and meaning, including the variable rhetorical effects that ensue from this relation. This also provides a pretext in which to examine the possible impact emoji design plays in the user-as-digital-rhetor's choice (Gray and Holmes Gray 2020: 4), which is especially empowering in developmental learning classrooms.

The field of analysis known as visual rhetoric (VR), which aims to analyze all kinds of visual images and texts as rhetorical structures, was historically an offshoot of both semiotics and of the psychology of visual thinking, defined as the capacity to extract meaning from visual images. The basic methodology of VR is traced back to semiotician Roland Barthes' pivotal 1964 article, "The Rhetoric of the Image," in which he showed how culturally shaped rhetorical meaning (metaphor, metonymy, catachresis, irony, and so on) can be embedded unconsciously in visual images. He used an ad for *Panzani* pasta to show how this unfolds – his analysis is worthwhile revisiting here in condensed summary form for the sake of illustration.

Barthes started his analysis by identifying different levels of meaning in the ad. First, there is the level of denotation consisting of the brand name and logo design. This has pure informational value – it allows viewers to recognize the pasta, should they desire to buy it. However, the name also works at a different connotative level, since it assigns an aura of "Italianicity" to the whole ad text. Connected to this is the symbolism of the tomato and the other ingredients, which are suggestive of Italian cuisine and its supposed superiority – a meaning reinforced by the caption ("*à l'italienne de luxe*"). This whole system of meanings constitutes a powerful unconscious rhetorical system, which he called a *code*, whereby the initial denotative reading of the ad is "noncoded" while the connotative one is "coded." He referred to the ways in which the images and caption led the viewer to the coded meaning as *anchorage*.

The key insight of VR for the present purposes is that emoji are similarly coded, albeit to different degrees, as they are "anchored" in the hybrid structure of a bimodal message (words and emoji). So, the image of a lion in, say, a message between two students discussing a professor, would bear coded rhetorical meaning, interpretable in terms of the historical connotations and figures of speech associated with lions. VR is showing that visual signs are de facto rhetorical objects and that, therefore, they can be used to influence and persuade people as effectively as classic rhetorical oratory, if not more so, but in a non-overt way, since visuality entails forming coded mental images. Phillip Yenawine (1997: 845) defines this process, in fact, as "the ability to find meaning in imagery":

> It involves a set of skills ranging from simple identification (naming what one sees) to complex interpretation on contextual, metaphoric and philosophical levels. Many aspects of cognition are called upon, such as personal association, questioning, speculating, analyzing, fact-finding, and categorizing. Objective understanding is the premise of much of this literacy, but subjective and affective aspects of knowing are equally important.

In line with general research in VR, emoji can be seen to affect people emotionally through the unconscious chain of coded connotations that they activate. It is this chain that has persuasive force. Hariman and Lucaites (2011) used this insight of VR to demonstrate how photographs are powerful visual texts capable of influencing public opinion on all kinds of social matters – recalling Barthes' own analysis of photography (Barthes 1977, 1981). Photos may seem to have many meanings, but given the context in which they occur (in a particular part of a newspaper, for example) they are anchored in such a way that viewers will be led to the intended message unconsciously. The same applies to emoji, as discussed, given that it is their placement in a hybrid text that activates the distributive process of meaning (discussed further in Chapter 7).

It should be mentioned that the pivotal work of the Belgian group μ, founded in 1967, has contributed significantly to our understanding of how VR affects us emotionally and cognitively. They refer to visual literacy as a critical function for understanding human thoughts and how they are formed. The logic of visual literacy is as inescapable as the rhetorical logic of verbal arguments. Group μ's 1970 publication, *A General Rhetoric*, reformulated classical rhetoric in visually based ways, classifying images according to their different rhetorical modalities. In their *Traité du signe visuel* (1992) they elaborated a "grammar of the image," defined in ways that are parallel to our notions of distributive and episodic structure. Each choice and allocation of an emoji thus represents a different "coding" of meaning that the user may want to portray to the interlocutor. This involves the conative function – the ability of a sign to influence a receiver in a particular way. In a study within the marketing field, but that nonetheless has relevance to the present discussion, Ge-Stadnyk and Gretzel (2018) studied the use of emoji on the part of social media influencers. Hundreds of posts by the top 200 Weibo influencers were collected by the researchers, which allowed them to develop a taxonomy of emoji-based rhetorical strategies aimed at encouraging specific responses in followers. The main finding was that emoji are processed unconsciously as highly suggestive of meaning, thus attracting followers to the object of interest that the emoji entails. In other words, the study corroborated Barthes' notion that images are coded for rhetorical meaning.

Aware of the rhetorical power of emoji, the marketing world has expanded the emoji code on its own, so as to get around the limitations imposed by the preset Unicode system. There are now custom branded emoji keyboards and sticker campaigns allowing brands to reach their consumers much more directly. To determine if such strategies are effective, Yakin and Eru (2017) measured the attitudes of advertisers and audiences toward emoji usage in social media marketing campaigns. The results indicated that emoji advertising was effective because of its ability to activate conative mechanisms. The researchers conclude as follows (Yakin and Eru 2017: 230):

> According to the results of the study, it has been concluded that emojis are effective for social advertising campaigns. Participants expressed that, usage of emojis in advertising campaigns is suitable for social campaigns. And using emojis in advertising campaigns explains the Project successfully. They expressed that the transmitted message of the campaign is informative and effective. And also participants expressed that these kinds of campaigns are attractive, creative and innovative.

Ge-Stadnyk and Gretzel (2018) found, moreover, that marketing-based emoji activate image-schematic processes that guide the reader to assign a range of controlled connotative-suggestive meanings through visual annotative structure. Without going into details of their work here, suffice it to say that the fact that "reading" the messages tends to leave viewers bewildered as to what they mean is due to the fact that they are not anchored in a word-based message.

All this has implications for language-literacy instruction since, as can be seen, emoji are inserted or combined to suggest a connection to other emoji in terms of referentiality, chronology, and narrativity – hence their episodic structure. Without the anchorage provided by words, the meaning cannot be constrained. For, example, how would one interpret "🏃 👰" or "⬅😔" (Ge-Stadnyk and Gretzel 2018)? The former can refer to a "runaway bride" and the latter to the action of "going to sleep." Both are coded for meaning, since they can only be understood by speakers of a language that possesses these combinations of concepts as idioms. Now, using such emoji forms in the classroom allows the students to decode their meaning on the basis of what they know. In fact, emoji can be used as devices to illustrate many of the devices of classical rhetoric, as part of a lesson on the relation between literacy practices and rhetorical discourses.

Epilogue

The use of emoji in various areas of education and in designing pedagogical practices constitutes an approach that envisions emoji literacy as part of an emergent, dynamic process shaped by technology, even though it could be ended by technology at some point. In bringing emoji into the classroom the same types of caveats that apply to the use of emoji in general apply even more strongly. First, there is the issue of cross-cultural variation and of the subjective interpretant, which must always be taken into account to avoid miscommunications and potential conflict. Second, there is the incompatibility of platforms, which might also lead to miscommunication. While many popular emoji keyboard apps, such as Bitmoji, make it easier for users to copy and paste an image into a message, it should always be kept in mind that emoji are platform-created characters with variant glyphic form. In effect, the variability factor in emoji usage is an increasingly relevant one. Yet, the very facility with which emoji can be transported into any educational context presents teachers with the opportunity to take advantage of a form of literacy that is not only in step with communications generally but also effective pedagogically, despite the provisos discussed here. The primary aim of incorporating emoji into education is to allow the classroom to adapt to the exigencies of users who have become accustomed to multimedia textualities, thus engaging students in creative ways so that their intellectual energies can be directed to learning necessary skills and content.

In a sense, the use of emoji in education parallels the suggestions by mathematics educators to use puzzles as creative devices for stimulating the interest of students in the discipline. In the last puzzle column that he wrote for *Scientific American*, the late well-known puzzle-maker Martin Gardner (1998) saw the use of puzzles "as a way to interest young students in the wonders of mathematics." The same observation can be applied to emoji, given that emoji can be utilized to introduce students in any discipline to the "wonders" of visual semiotics in expressing and encoding knowledge. These devices immerse students cognitively into the conceptual system of the discipline being taught through the processes connected to visuality. The benefits that this may bring about are similar to the benefits of using puzzles in a different domain – foreign language teaching. McDonald (2007: 149) summarizes these benefits as follows:

> The general advantages of using logic puzzles are that they can be both mentally challenging and fun for students while producing numerous pedagogical benefits. These benefits are believed to include an increased exposure to vocabulary presented in specific contexts with a distinct focus on comprehending meaning, a heightened mental engagement with the key vocabulary at a deep level of processing, and the fostering of inference skills and the ability to guess meaning from context, all in a relatively brief amount of class time. Furthermore, logic puzzles offer a great deal of adaptability in exactly how they are utilized in class. Ultimately, it can be concluded that logic puzzles should be explored more thoroughly for their potential benefits to classroom teaching and the learning of foreign languages.

The kinds of activities that emoji make possible within the classroom, some of which have been discussed in this chapter, may also set in motion bimodal learning (Chapter 2), activating the flow of learning from the R-Mode to the L-Mode. This is in line with the notion of conceptual blending, developed by Gilles Fauconnier and Mark Turner (2002) – a process that underlies novel ideas via the blending of previously-acquired or familiar concepts and procedures. As Vespoor (2008: 23) has aptly pointed out, this type of approach is effective because it allows for the separate aspects of a learning task to become blended in a way that favors meaning-based understanding:

> Traditionally language has been viewed as an autonomous system, separate from other cognitive and social abilities. In this view, the language system operates under a set of arbitrary and unmotivated rules and properties and the various subcomponents of the language system such as syntax, morphology, and lexis are independent of each other. The approach to language learning that accompanies this view of language emphasizes the need for the learner to learn vocabulary items separately, master the grammar rules and memorize their exceptions. A radically different view of the language system is found in a cognitive linguistic approach. Cognitive Linguistics (CL) is based on the assumption that meaning is embodied and attempts to explain facts about language in terms of other properties and mechanisms of the human mind and body.

Emoji involve an inner modeling process that is independent of the specific categories of a language but can be anchored to it – as such, it allows the student to enter into the cognitive space of a discipline without reliance on the categories of a language in any formal way. The effectiveness of this general bimodal feature of learning has been corroborated by several studies. For example, McCrea and Robinson (2011) found that visually based pedagogical devices activated "predominately right frontoparietal networks involved in visual working memory" at the same time that they involved "the integrity of the left temporoparietal junction." Fallows and Hilsabeck (2012: 932) found that such devices were not exclusively dependent on visual processing, but depended as well on verbal and other processes, concluding that "memory, mental flexibility, processing speed, and language abilities also contribute to successful performance of the task."

In sum, the incorporation of emoji and other multimedia devices into education does not sever the flow of educational history, but rather shapes its direction in sync with technological changes. If some object becomes obsolete, such as the typewriter, then it is eliminated from everyday usage but not forgotten, since typewriter keyboards became computer keyboards. Indeed, the first PCs were called "word processors," since they were seen as simply extending the functions of typewriters, adding the capacity for automatic correction and memory storage within the device itself. So, what changed was not the "word," as such, but the "technology of the word." Digital signs, texts, and codes do not sever their structural ties with signs in general; they repackage them in new technological ways, but in so doing, they engender novel ways of representing the world – and these have definite implications for understanding who we are and where we are headed. This is what McLuhan intended with his now famous phrase "the medium is the message," which encapsulates the fact that the technological media we use for constructing and communicating information shapes the content of that information. As these technologies change, so too does our understanding of information. McLuhan (1964: 22–23) put it succinctly as follows:

> The medium is the message. This is merely to say that the personal and social consequences of any medium – that is, of any extension of ourselves – result from the new scale that is introduced into our affairs by each extension of ourselves, or by any new technology.

Digital signs such as emoji exist everywhere today. As such, they present new problems of analysis for what they mean, how they can be used, and what implications they bear for the future of literacy and communication more generally. They are sometimes seen as having impoverished how we write and think. But, even if this were so (which we believe it is not), then, as McLuhan emphasized, we will always find ways to solve problems of meaning. As he facetiously put it: "Instead of scurrying into a corner and wailing about what media are doing to us, one should charge straight ahead and kick them in the electrodes" (McLuhan 1960: 148). Technology is neither good nor bad; it is what we make of it. When asked about this very idea, McLuhan (1987: 300) responded insightfully as follows:

> My main theme is the extension of the nervous system in the electric age, and thus, the complete break with five thousand years of mechanical technology. This I state over and over again. I do not say whether it is a good or bad thing. To do so would be meaningless and arrogant.

The classroom of the future, as McLuhan predicted in 1960, would be a technologically shaped one that is designed to open up the learning experience beyond the constrained environment of the traditional "walled-in" classroom. In the era of the Internet and social media this has certainly come about, as students and teachers alike communicate among themselves and with others through cyberspace on a routine basis. But in order for the new learning-teaching environment to make sense, many of the pedagogical practices of the traditional walled-in classroom must also be constantly retrieved in various ways. So, in the case of literacy training, the retrieval occurs through semioliteracy training, which takes into account the different sign modalities and the different media (verbal and nonverbal) used to construct meanings.

Technologies are not revolutionary on a social level; they are evolutionary, linking the various phases of the past into a flow that originated through and shaped by previous technological changes. Change in human systems is thus organic. This means that new educational methods have not degraded teaching that used print materials, but rather have retrieved them organically. As McLuhan (1964: 240) remarked: "New media are new archetypes, at first disguised as degradations of older media." The advent of "classrooms without walls" means that students, teachers, and others are connected constantly, being no longer restricted by the time and space constraints of the physical classroom. McLuhan (1960: 3) summarized this situation as follows:

> These new developments, under quiet analytic survey, point to a basic strategy of culture for the classroom. When the printed book first appeared, it threatened the oral procedures of teaching and created the classroom as we now know it. Instead of making his own text, his own dictionary, his own grammar, the student started out with these tools. He could study not one but several languages. Today these new media threaten, instead to merely reinforce, the procedures of this traditional classroom. It's customary to answer this threat with denunciations of the unfortunate character and effect of movies and TV, just as the comic book was feared and scorned and rejected from the classroom. Its good and bad features in form and content, when carefully set beside other kinds of art and narrative, could have become a major asset to the teacher.

It is truly remarkable that emoji appeared in 1999 as a set of 176 symbols that were meant to convey visually-compacted information about the weather, traffic, technology and time. Today, they convey all kinds of meanings across languages, cultures, lifestyles, and professions. As we have argued here, while emoji look like cute, harmless visual signs, they could mean something entirely different to individuals in different areas of the world and individuals of different ages. The younger generation is typically the one that initiates and uses the changes in emoji that bear relevance to how we think and even learn today. Educators con no longer avoid them, at least at the present time, otherwise they not only risk losing the opportunity to profit from what students bring to the learning situation, but also remain unaware of the many modalities of meaning that this often complex ever-changing code entails.

7 Implications and Applications

Prologue

Some scholars now consider emoji to be a new universal language – a kind of "pop Esperanto" that people use worldwide, largely agreeing on what the core lexicon of emoji signs covers or, at least, intends to cover. However, different countries and cultures have their own preferred emoji, often with varying meanings. But it is also true that the overall intent of emoji use is to facilitate global village communications via the visuality aspect of emoji signs. As descendants of emoticons, born in 1982 out of the need to minimize digital miscommunications, by 1999 a Japanese wireless mobile company developed the technology needed to generate emoji. This made character limits more manageable. The initial set included 172 emoji icons created to simplify multimedia messaging. By 2011, computer companies adopted the emoji phenomenon after its increasingly widening popularity, making keyboards and apps with emoji characters available throughout the world. As mentioned several times, as a result of the technology, the ways in which people communicate in writing and how they extract meaning from texts has moved away from the pattern of representing and interpreting them in the print age.

Another consequence of the technology has been that emoji have become part of their own literacy, migrating to various areas of digital communications, such as the two that have been the target of interest in this book – healthcare and education. The incorporation of emoji into these areas, however, has yet to become a stable institutionalized practice. The studies conducted by the authors of this book point directly to the viability and feasibility of such systematic institutionalization. The reason for connecting emoji use in healthcare and education is the fact that both involve the public in direct ways, and both entail the need to make communications inclusive and highly comprehensible. In this final chapter, we will go over the main ideas that have emerged from the research, bolstered by our analysis of the relevant literature. As we have argued throughout, these can be used as starting points to develop emoji-based communicative practices in both healthcare and education. The results of the "applied emoji research" discussed here have several implications at the theoretical and even socio-philosophical levels. These include: implications for emoji theory and for the future of writing and communication in an ever-expanding age of artificial intelligence.

The diffusion of emoji in all areas of everyday communicative-expressive life is now a fact. The domains of healthcare and education are slowly catching up to this trend. As our research has shown, emoji pedagogy, when applied to learning environments in a contextualized way, enhances learning for students regardless of their backgrounds, given that the emoji lexicon is understandable to virtually everyone. This is a major psychological element of emoji use in practical situations. For example, Maud Donga (2019), an instructor at a Dutch university for applied sciences, studied the value of emoji in education, corroborating the findings and patterns of learning discussed in previous chapters. Donga found that by integrating emoji with written words in the classroom to carry out specific tasks (such as reading and writing), students displayed a spontaneous shift from information-processing of classroom input to the assigning of meaning to it intuitively, which reinforces not only the learning process *in actu* but also retention. Donga concluded that it is the unconscious absorption of a concept via the visuality of emoji that makes what we call here emoji pedagogy effective, especially given the fact that it is intrinsic to how students themselves communicate outside the classroom.

Implications for Emoji Theory

The research studies discussed in this book have borne a number of concrete implications for emoji theory in general. The advent of emoji indicates that there are now two main modes of informal writing with their own specific semiotic forms – verbal (based on script) and visual (based on emoji in particular). A word written with alphabet characters, as mentioned several times, is designed to represent its phonemic structure, aiming to match the spoken word in written form. On the other hand, emoji cannot be broken down in the same way as alphabetic words; they are holistic visual signs that stand for referents directly. In most digital texts, emoji are used in tandem with written words, producing a hybrid writing code, which allows interlocutors to use both the alphabet and the emoji code in tandem to create messages that enfold iconic, indexical, and symbolic features. As discussed, a facial emoji, for instance, is essentially an icon; an arrow emoji, which points to something, is an index; and a raised thumb emoji is a symbol, since it has different meanings according to culture.

Above all else, as part of an informal mode of expression, emoji perform specific semiotic and discursive functions, complementing, supplementing, and annotating verbal message content. They cannot replace verbal explication in areas that are knowledge-seeking, such as science and mathematics (and others), which involve the systematic study of the structure and behavior of the physical and natural world and the testing of theories against the evidence obtained. In these fields, emoji can be used heuristically to relay complex scientific knowledge to nonscientists, such as in clinician–patient interactions; but they would have no discernible function in the elaboration of scientific facts, as such. Their primary communicative contexts are SMS messages, emails, tweets, and the like. In highly formal contexts (such as science, philosophy, mathematics), emoji, as holistic signs, do not have the ability to relay the precise information that may be required, and thus are not replacements for other kinds of visual devices used formally, such as diagrams and charts. Emoji, therefore, have a time and a place. Some do depict science, technology, and even reading. These have, as mentioned, a heuristic function. Of course, scientists and scholars, as we have seen, can also employ emoji while in communication with their network of peers. But this is, clearly, a subjective function of science.

Technology

Emoji have been typically described as pictographs at various levels of representation, from the purely iconic one to those that involve abstractions, assuming, more precisely, ideographic qualities (Chapter 1). But emoji are not really pictographs, in the historical sense of the term; they are prefabricated visual signs that can be selected from a keyboard or app, much like any other kind of writing character. For this reason, some have preferred to characterize them as similar to the public signs that are put in places to indicate something (danger, prohibition to enter somewhere, etc.), which are also language-independent and designed to have a fixed set of universally understandable meanings. However, unlike such static sign forms, emoji meanings cannot be pinned down so easily; moreover, they can be used with other types of signs, including in combinations with other emoji, allowing for the expression of a vast array of meanings.

It is relevant to note that the earliest pictographs were not standardized picture words, as such; they were mainly sketches suggesting referents, as is evident in the carvings and paintings on roofs and walls of ancient caves (Schmandt-Besserat 1978, 1992). Emoji are also suggestive signs, having eclipsed their initial definition as picture words via constant usage in all kinds of communicative contexts. They have been made possible by technology, not through the usual channels of linguistic evolution, that is, through the process by which different words and other verbal structures have developed and diversified from earlier forms in the history of a language (or writing system). The changes that are presently occurring in emoji are due to innovations in technology and via new forms invented daily by institutions such as Unicode to keep up with demands for new emoji signs, as well as to emerging needs of interlocutors as they use them routinely.

Emoji have thus come forward as prefabricated, mass-produced artifacts intended to allow interaction in the global village to be as fluid as possible, given the diversity of languages within it. As our own studies showed, in line with the general findings, emoji signs do indeed allow members of different cultures to participate in the exchange of messages, allowing them to feel equal participants in these exchanges, even if problems of interpretation arise constantly in the realm of visual meaning. But emoji are not mere conveyors of information through the visual channel; they have the ability to influence interlocutors via the "feeling states" they encode and convey, rather than the "thinking states" that words entail. As Aldous Huxley (1942: 82) so perceptively remarked about visual communication in general, this is likely what makes emoji so powerful as semiotic artifacts:

> Within your visual communication there will inevitably be some information or meaning beyond the image itself for the person seeing to find. This makes visual communication a very powerful tool, by influencing what people see, you influence what they know, and by influencing what they know you further influence what they see.

In a pertinent neuropsychological study, Paggio and Tse (2022) looked at how emoji are processed in contrast to written words, finding that their interpretation is in fact processed differently from words, involving complexity of decipherment. The researchers investigated how individuals reacted to emoji using an eye tracking method. They found that: (1) emoji are more difficult to process than words; and (2) that their processing is subject to ambiguity factors. Overall, this implies that emoji are more than picture words, projecting face-to-face conversational devices onto the screen in a visual way. Access to emoji meaning is more complex than what the creators thought would emerge with these new signs. Nonredundant emoji in particular are more difficult to integrate in the processing of sentences than the equivalent words, or emoji used in a redundant (purely descriptive) way. As the researchers concluded, in line with our own findings and observations, "emoji may not always be as immediate and easy to process for readers in spite of their popularity."

Communicative Functions

The general linguistic research on emoji has focused, by and large, on the communicative functions that these visual signs seem to bear. However, assigning a communicative function to an emoji, or set of emoji (such as the facial ones), cannot be detached from considering its distributional and annotative features. In effect, emoji perform semiotic and discursive functions in tandem, and the latter are likely derived from the former. A smiley face may indeed be an utterance opener (similar to "Hi"), but it also imbues the entire text with its sentiment and thus might affect the distribution and selection of subsequent signs, much like the elements in a painting cohere meaningfully.

The Jakobsonian functions can be enlisted to explain emoji use in a general way – including the emotive, conative, poetic, phatic, and metalingual functions. The emotive function is a key one in emoji use, as we also discovered in our research projects. In a healthcare situation, as we saw, the provider can use appropriate emoji in a digital communication with patients to encourage or convince them of the need to follow a prescribed therapy. This is accomplished by the very nature of emoji as feeling-based structures with the inbuilt capacity to open up the channels of understanding in an unconscious empathic way (Chapters 4 and 5). This very same function applies to literacy training, as we also saw especially with developmental students (Chapter 2). On the other side of emotivity is conativity, that is, the actual ability of an emoji-structured message to influence receivers, especially the capacity to grab their attention effectively. The poetic function implies the ability of emoji to deliver meaning in rhetorically effective ways, as in poetry. The phatic aspects of emoji-based interaction surfaced in many of the studies examined here, including our own. This is a bonding function, found typically in opening and closing protocols in conversations, via emoji such as smiley faces, hearts, and the like. More generally, however, the use of emoji throughout a digital conversation entails phatic communion, as Malinowski (1922) called it; that is, their use tends to lubricate the conversation in a positive way. Finally, as our foray into the educational domain has made clear to us, emoji also have a metalingual function, making some abstract concept in, say, an English or mathematics class more understandable, since it involves using the visual channel to present information that is otherwise complex or abstract, no matter the level of learning involved.

The above functions are shaped by contextual factors, which affect emoji meanings, typically refining them in specific ways (culturally, psychologically, socially, etc.). In hybrid writing, which involves the blending of verbal and visual signs intended to express some message or intent in tandem, different contextual cues associated with each modality are involved, thus expanding Michael Halliday's (1985) notion of systemic grammar, whereby the parts of speech are analyzed in terms of text-governed structures, not grammatical ones in themselves. Emoji are similarly text-governed signs, which, together with words, are sensitive to the contextual cues that oscillate between verbal and visual dimensions. In practice this implies that emoji are not inserted in digital messages just to reinforce the meaning or to project nonverbal cues onto the text, but rather to assume contextualized functions in tandem with words.

Within a systemic framework, therefore, emoji are inserted at points in a message that are sensitive to the relevance and quality of the content and pertinent to the implicit protocols of a conversation. Below are a few illustrative examples, which indicate how emoji function within a systemic textual grammar.

- *Turn-taking*. When people are involved in a conversation, they do not talk all at the same time – one person speaks, and then another person can follow. A turn becomes evident through certain forms that interlocutors recognize and count on. These allow speakers to predict when someone is finished so that others can speak, so as to minimize both overlap and silence. Examples of turn-taking (or more precisely turn-requesting) emoji inserted in digital conversations are the following – placed at points where intervention is desired. Note that these are not just simulated vocal or gestural signals projected onto the digital screen; rather, they portray the gestures in ways that involve sentiment as well, as can be seen by the expression on the facial emoji:

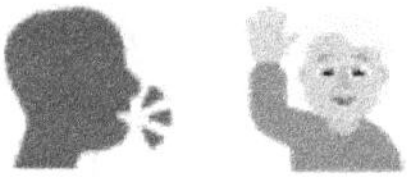

- *Commentary.* Emoji are sometimes placed in locations to provide commentary on an ongoing interaction. The following, for example, mean respectively, "I'm listening but not really able to focus" and "I won't say a word!" simulating counterpart physical gestures used in face-to-face communication, but adding semantic nuances that are not normally found in gestural signals (such as those that characterize humor and bafflement). In effect, the emoji assume semiotic and discursive functions at the same time, not independently:

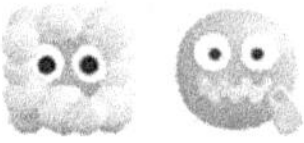

- *Expansion.* Emoji are sometimes placed in locations where interlocutors wish to expand upon something or want the other interlocutor to expand on what was intended. Examples include the two below, which mean respectively "I don't understand" (simulating the relevant gesture) and sarcastically, "Yeah, right!" Again, both emoji involve more than gestural resemblance; they make a humorous commentary on the gesture and situation itself:

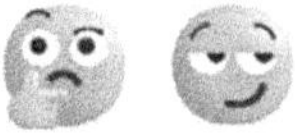

- *Repair*. This type of emoji allows interlocutors to deal with problems of understanding, such as repairing the negative effects of some comment. Below are two examples, meaning respectively "I'm sorry" (simulating the corresponding facial expression) and "I made a mistake" (imitating the relevant hand gesture). As above, however, these are not just simulative gestural signs; they involve embedded annotations that convey sentiments of specific kinds (such as sadness or regret):

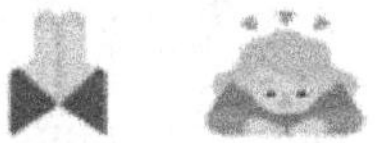

- *Reactions*. Some emoji indicate what reactions are evoked on basis of the content of a message. Examples include the following, meaning respectively "I'm losing my temper" (or, "I'm coming to the end of my patience") and "I am angry," which are self-explanatory as to their semiotic effects:

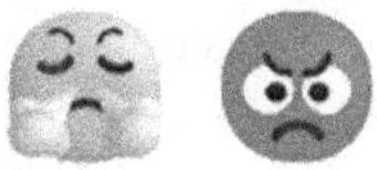

These are examples of how emoji placement is text-governed and thus reflective of an expanded systemic grammar. To cite Halliday (1985: 15), such uses can be seen to add to the "network of systems, or interrelated sets of options for making meaning." The blending of emoji functions with words in texts reveals what Halliday calls the multidimensional architecture of language.

The use of emoji to convey negative sentiments, and even hate (discussed below), merits special attention, given the possibility that such usage could creep into interactions (surreptitiously) in healthcare and educational settings. In a special 2020 issue of *Social Semiotics*, the focus of the contributions was, in fact, on examining the use of emoji to convey aggression and hate, rather than positive sentiments (for example, Benavides-Vanegas 2020; Cheng, Yuxiu, and Li 2020; Matulewska and Gwiazdowicz 2020). As Wagner, Marusek, and Yu (2020) emphasized in that issue, the hidden power of emoji communication is that it can "fundamentally alter the exchange of emotion [because] images and signs that depict feelings have replaced the nuanced selection of the right words and phrases." It is this dimension of emoji usage that can lead to, or elicit, all kinds of aggressive meanings. As the authors surmise: "Across the globe, the expressive range of human emotion through the static ideogram of the emoji, or emoticon, presents an increasing challenge for the visually immediate, non-verbal exchange of capricious emotive communication."

The aggression sentiment is signaled often by the repetition of specific emoji, such as a sequence of gun emoji in a threatening message (🔫 🔫 🔫 🔫), as Wagner and Yu (2021) pointed out in a subsequent study:

> The more they multiply them in writing, the more the intensity is getting reinforced. This emotional load, which could be positive, negative or even aggressive, is therefore one of the verbal triggers in bashing.

So, while the range of communicative functions emoji typically revolve around the conveyance of positivity, there is always the potential for communicating aggression, conflict, and even hate. Moreover, ambiguity, variability, and contrastive meanings are always present factors in emoji discourse. So, despite the original objective of creating a visual Esperanto for culture-neutral, nonaggressive communication, the use of emoji for various subjective intents cannot be curtailed. Taming negativity in communicative systems is not exclusive to emoji use, but the need to ensure that it does not occur in education in general is a major goal of a putative "applied emojistics," as it can be called, in parallel to applied linguistics. By identifying, investigating, and offering solutions to communication-related problems, applied emojistics can play a role in decoding the meanings behind everyday interactions.

Annotation

The foregoing discussion brings us to a major finding of our own research (which parallels other research studies) – namely, that a central feature of emoji use is its capacity to allow users to provide annotative perspectives to a message. Even the use of a smiley face in response to some statement is annotative in the sense that it reveals in a visual way what the interlocutor is thinking or feeling, rather than just fulfilling a communicative function or subserving some turn-taking response. Annotation also allows the user to make something clear or understandable, which, as we saw in the healthcare world, is a key use of emoji, allowing, for instance, medical doctors to explain symptoms to patients, without the need to use technical terms that might activate a sense of foreboding in the patient. Annotation is a way to establish a common ground between interlocutors with different levels of knowledge, or else to add perspective to the emoji sign as it occurs in specific locations. The value of annotation in the medical field has been studied during the pandemic (as mentioned previously), whereby teleconsultations became loci for emoji use – allowing doctors to convey messages visually and effectively during a crisis.

All uses of emoji bear some intent, not just information or some communicative protocol, providing nuances in meaning that shape the overall effect of a message. They are not substitutions of written forms (picture words) or visually artifactual projections of nonverbal signals onto the screen; rather, they provide user perspectives, even when the function is a nonverbal one. So, for example, the smiley-based commentary emoji above  is not just a simulated facial microexpression, but an annotative sign as well – adding nuances including concern or bewilderment. While this occurs in face-to-face communication, in the emoji form it is part and parcel of the form itself, not a semiotic option. This can, of course, also be conveyed through words and stylistic modulations, but it is much easier to do so by selecting an emoji, which comes already designed to convey such nuances (wittingly or not). So, the smiley emoji can be used to convey irony in a conflictual message, and the tears with joy one can communicate consternation in the context of contradictory information in a message. In other words, the emoji are not communicatively tagged pictograms; they allow interlocutors to control the intent of discourse, adding "silent commentary" to a message, to use a phrase introduced by anthropologist Edward T. Hall (1959).

As Pereira-Kohatsu, Quijano-Sánchez, Liberatore, and Camacho-Collados (2019: 4564) have also noted, the annotative functions of emoji, from reinforcing the meaning of a message to even subverting it, are constantly at play in emoji use in a distinctive way with respect to any counterparts in verbal, prosodic, or gestural communication:

> Emoji can be used as a supplemental modality to clarify the intended sense of an ambiguous message, attach sentiment to a message, or subvert the original meaning of the text entirely in ways a word could not. Emoji carry meaning on their own, and possess compositionality allowing for more nuanced semantics through multi-emoji phrases.

In sum, the pragmatic (communicative) functions overlap constantly with the annotative ones. Like real-world facial microexpressions, emoji have indeed assumed many of the thoughts and feelings that these suggest, but they add more to these via annotation. Phatic speech is a crucial aspect of bonding rituals and a means for putting forth what the sociologist Erving Goffman (1959) termed a "positive social face" during interactional situations. So, a smiley emoji used at the beginning of a text message similarly provides a positive social face, but it goes beyond the social protocol by imbuing the tone of the message with positivity, thus ensuring that bonding between the interlocutors is maintained. An emoji put at the end of a message often summarizes the content of that message, thus leaving a kind of annotative fingerprint on the tone. An end-of-message ironic face emoji, for example, may encapsulate the satirical intent of the message, keeping the message fluid nonetheless, which would be much more difficult to do with ironic or sarcastic words.

Now, while an addresser may select a facial emoji with a specific intent, it may not achieve the elicitation of the same feeling or sense in the addressee. A key study by Ma, Liu, Wang, and Vosiughi (2020) has shed significant light on this annotative-conative aspect of emoji use. While the researchers used the term "annotation" in reference to providing prompts to an AI software (Transformer) in order to track sentiment use in digital texts, the findings have concrete implications for emoji theory, at least in this domain. As they aptly observe: "Predicting the proper emojis associated with text provides a way to summarize the text accurately," even though, in itself, "one single emoji cannot fully cover the theme of a piece of text." Goffman (1963) referred to the amalgam of annotative sense with overall communicative intent as a "co-presence" in all kinds of messages, so that the subjective and the objective (informational) aspects of communication merge systemically, unlike information exchanges in all other species.

Semantic and Episodic Processing

Competence in using emoji involves the ability to map textual sequences against visual episodes, as in a comic book or a children's illustrated story. As an example of how this might unfold in a specific way, consider a specific text message, which was a well-known meme in Internet culture found on many public domain websites. The intent of the text is actually enunciated at the top in words – "Dude, let's rob a bank." The emoji are arranged in an episodic dialogical form, laid out from top to bottom. The top line portrays the opening sequence of events laid out in temporal order: gun (the weapon for robbing the bank) + money bag (the booty that results from the robbery) + car (the escape vehicle). The line below is the response by the interlocutor's potential partner. It shows a grinning face emoji suggesting that the respondent is unsure about the outcome of the robbery. The third line (from the first interlocutor) shows an admittance of the danger, with relevant emoji-simulated episodes of what might happen next – namely, police cars will be summoned to the scene, to which the partner responds with a frowning face, conveying a feeling of anxiety. The fifth line then portrays the likely scenario that will unfold: guns (shooting that will take place between the robbers and the police) + fire truck + ambulance (indicating the usual order of the arrival of these emergency vehicles, suggesting a possibility of injury). The final query – "So that's a no then?" – implies the denouement to the episodes, much like in a story. Now, the use of emoji in some (perhaps many) digital communications involves a similar marking of episodes in the content of a message. As such, the "emoji grammar" might best be called an "episodic grammar."

In the decipherment of emoji episodic sequences or structure in general, the annotative dimension always comes into play. Consider the gun emoji in the text message above. On its own, it represents a specific referent – a weapon with a particular form. But when used in combination with the other signs it takes on annotative, figuratively based meanings. So, even in the text it elicits the senses of "danger," "weapon of choice in robberies," "death," "violence," and so on. The intent of a text will constrain the range of such meanings, of course; but these cannot be totally controlled, even in texts such as the one above, which could be taken as a satirical dialogue, rather than a serious one. In any case, emoji, like the images in comic books, clearly have an episodic function, visually depicting the events or relevant aspects of a narrative – a finding that came out as well in our research on healthcare communications (Chapter 4). The annotative-metaphorical meanings that can be assigned to episodes in a text reveal a semantic function, rather than a purely communicative one.

In the psychological literature, episodic memory is a category of long-term memory that involves the recollection of specific events, situations, and experiences. This subsystem of memory is typically projected through emoji onto a text, such as the one discussed earlier. In a text where the interlocutors are reminiscing about, say, their college days together, emoji representing college mascots (such as animal emoji), recollections of actual classes (with emoji of professor figures, classrooms, etc.), and the like will tend to be allocated to specific locations in the message by both interlocutors. These visually provide a sense of personal and shared history, allowing the interlocutors to visually encapsulate experiences that helped shape their lives. As mentioned, the term episodic memory was first introduced by Endel Tulving in 1972 to distinguish between remembering events from the past (episodic memory) and recalling factual information, generally through words (semantic memory). Episodic sign structures allow for the recounting of events in texts that involve some aspect of autobiography or else project autobiographical experiences onto the annotation of a particular message. In effect, episodic grammar allows interlocutors to bring autobiography to bear on a situation, as well as allowing for an imaginative reconstruction of episodes from the past. If the digital interaction involves autobiographical experiences, then the emoji selected to fill in certain spots in a message might include, say, marriage, first car, or job emoji. Among other episodic functions the following are worth noting here (Conway 2009):

(1) An episodic emoji, such as a college mascot, is a visual record of some experienced event that is shared with the interlocutor, because the interlocutor either was part of the event or else is informed about it as meaningful. It implies an annotative-affective projection of memory, which augments the emotive and conative functions considerably.
(2) An episodic emoji is often a memento. So, for instance, the emoji of a classic automobile might represent a memento of one's first experience with driving.
(3) The processing of episodic emoji is akin to how we read comic books, whereby the image and the text become integrated into an overall system of bimodal understanding (as it has been called in this book).
(4) Episodic emoji convey a subjective perspective. The car emoji, for instance, conveys a perspective on both the person's understanding of the cultural-social aspects of driving and the autobiographical importance of the automobile to the interlocutor.

(5) Episodic emoji highlight the role of the imagination in recalling events or bringing episodes that bear autobiographical meaning into a discourse.
(6) Overall, episodic emoji constitute elements in an ongoing narrative of self-hood intended to evoke empathy on the part of the receiver. We witnessed this in several of the texts used in the healthcare education experiment (Chapter 4), which showed how reactions to autobiographical messages evoked empathy for the writer.
(7) In sum, episodic emoji make autobiographical meaning a constant factor in the layout of emoji in a text, either explicitly or implicitly.

Researchers have found that episodic memory is often interdependent with semantic memory (Kan, Alexander and Verfaillie 2009). On learning tasks, participants performed better when new information was aligned with prior knowledge, suggesting that semantic knowledge integrated with episodic knowledge provides a framework for processing novel content, as we ourselves witnessed in both experiments (Chapters 2 and 4), whereby, for example, the students in the developmental literacy class brought their backgrounds into the classroom spontaneously via episodic emoji usage, which allowed for its coordination with the goals of a particular lesson.

As an aside, the research has shown that aging and neurodegenerative diseases take an extreme toll on episodic memory – a notable decline in the ability to retrieve this kind of memory is among the first signs of Alzheimer's disease. This suggests that emoji may play a role in such cases as part of a therapeutic approach, which in turn suggests a path for future research. Other conditions such as dissociative disorders and Parkinson's disease also involve deficits in episodic memory functions, as does traumatic brain injury, such as a concussion. Again, the use of emoji in a therapeutic way may bear fruit, and thus requires further investigation. A significant study by Chatzichristos et al. (2020) actually confirmed our therapeutic hypothesis. The researchers presented evidence of the effect of emoji on memory retrieval through an fMRI study. Successive stimuli were presented to the participants, containing words with intense emotional content combined with emoji, with either congruent or incongruent emotive content. They were asked to recall a memory related to the stimuli. The reaction times showed that emotional incongruity among word + emoji combinations led to longer reaction times in memory retrieval compared to congruent combinations. The fMRI data showed, moreover, that word + emoji combinations activated Broca's area in both hemispheres, the supplementary motor area, and the inferior prefrontal cortex. Furthermore, when compared to pseudowords, the word + emoji combinations activated Broca's area in the left hemisphere, the amygdala, the right temporal lobe, and several frontal regions. Translating this finding in terms of bimodality theory, it can be seen that it is R-Mode activation that contributes to retrieval of memory via emoji, which is, clearly, a significant finding.

In another study, Clough et al. (2023) studied facial emotion recognition deficits after moderate–severe traumatic brain injury. The researchers examined whether emotion recognition deficits extended to the facial expressions depicted by emoji. Fifty-one individuals viewed photos of human faces and emoji faces, selecting the best-fitting label from a set of basic emotions. Participants did not significantly differ from neurotypical peers in overall emotion labeling accuracy. Both groups had poorer labeling accuracy for emoji compared to faces. Participants (but not neurotypical peers) had poorer accuracy for labeling social emotions depicted by emoji compared to basic emotions depicted by emoji. This is a contrastive finding that, clearly, requires future work.

Image Schemas

As discussed previously, any emoji can be described as an image schema, in the sense used both in cognitive linguistics as the mental outline that motivates metaphorical speech (Lakoff and Johnson 1980, 1999), and more broadly as the visual encoding of experiences in the form of mental imagery in schematic form. Image schema theory is useful in explaining the actual form of an emoji and how it relates to the inner images that it evokes. The opposite is also true – that is, an emoji used in a text can often trigger the appropriate schema in the brain that leads to its selection. So, a smiley face is, fundamentally, a schematic face, in this sense, constructed with the bare outline features of faces. It thus represents the face in its essential image-schematic form.

The range of potential image schemas that can be transferred to emoji form is constrained by actual physical and affective experiences and everyday events. It is the image-schematic structure of emoji speech that leaves the signs open to interpretation – as meanings are assigned to the schemas in context. This actually shows a metonymic function of emoji, revealing a part–whole reasoning process, such as the placement of the emoji of an automobile in a text in which pollution and climate change are the main themes at strategic locations. Irony, too, is based on the schematic form of an emoji, as we saw earlier with the facial commentary emoji, which gives satirical nuances a concrete visual form.

Distributional Semantics

A key feature of emoji usage is its distributional structure, whereby the meaning of a specific emoji can become a thematic element throughout the message – that is, it can affect the choice and meanings of other (subsequent emoji) in a text. This is a more specific term for Halliday's systemic (text-governed) analysis, expanding it into the visual realm. A simple example would be the use of a smiley face emoji at the beginning of a text that is designed to imbue the entire message with a positive sentiment, reinforced by emoji interspersed throughout the content that distribute the positivity throughout. The smiley thus provides the interpretive frame for imbuing the tone of the entire message with positivity, ensuring that a phatic bond between interlocutors is established. Of course, if a different kind of sentiment is intended, then the distribution of that sentiment ensues in a parallel way. Consider a well-known emoji text message on the Internet where a salutation protocol unfolds in an English-speaking ambiance.

The message starts with several portrait emoji – emoji that identify the addresser (male face, suit and tie, pants, business shoes, briefcase). The female addressee is identified with corresponding portraiture schemas (female face, dress, shoes, and welcoming kiss). The female interlocutor signs the message not with her name, but with a baby emoji that represents, suggestively, their child, followed by child talk ("Da Da"). This salutation protocol alludes to a nuclear family life as the one in which the interlocutors exist. This meaning is distributed via the emoji in sequence, which visually produce a composite picture of the type of family life that the text conveys. This distributive feature clearly overlaps with the autobiographical episodic one. This shows that emoji grammar is not a replica of linguistic grammar with visual symbols; it has episodic-distributional structure, much like a comic book.

The underlying strategy by which an interlocutor shapes the information content of a message via emoji distribution is often designed to take receivers "into the situation" to which senders apparently want to draw attention. This is virtually synonymous with what Goodwin and Goodwin (1992: 181) have designated "assessments," that is, strategies that "provide participants with resources for displaying evaluations of events and people in ways that are relevant to larger projects that they are engaged in." It bears witness to the fact that individual motivations and feelings, recollections, priorities, beliefs, and the like undergird the structuring of speech acts.

Register

Throughout this book, the claim has been made that emoji are not designed to convey register in the usual sense, although they are employed to signal aspects of politeness in various ways (as discussed). Verbal interactions vary in socially based ways to conform to the backgrounds and level of familiarity of the speakers. The two main general registers are formal and informal – modes of speaking or writing that are designed to match the social formality of a situation. Emoji, by their very nature, are part of informal discourse. However, they do not infringe on the polite tone in interactions that involve differential roles, such as in physician–patient interactions. The overall tone of such interactions is generally quasi-formalistic and polite. The insertion of emoji in such interactions, as we saw previously, does not impugn the politeness tone, but rather provides an intermittent break from the formal register, injecting a sense of empathy within it that gives the text a duality that is unique in writing and general communicative practices, which can be simplified as follows: written text = politeness tone, emoji insertions = empathic tone. This duality guarantees that one would avoid an ironic or vulgar emoji, intended for humor (such as the poop emoji), because it would impugn the overall politeness tone of the interaction.

The primary reason why emoji have not been constructed to mark distinctions in register may well be the initial intent of creating them to cross all cultural-social spheres so as to unite people in a common visual language, unmarked by the sociolinguistic distinctions of verbal language. They are attempts to install a sense of phatic communion throughout the global village, even though the results have not borne this out, as discussed. Phatic communion entails verbal exchanges that have bonding social functions and are thus mainly formulaic in this sense. When we greet someone with "How are you?" we hardly expect a medical report, as would a doctor. The function of that statement is simply to make contact. This type of social bonding occurs via specific speech formulas and in ritualistic contexts that guide their implementation. In the global village, one of the functions of emoji is to make the same kind of social bonding possible, despite the constant possibility of misinterpretation. Emoji may thus help new acquaintances to explore and categorize each other's social position or even opinions about common themes (politics, art, entertainment, etc.). They are social lubricants that help people feel more comfortable in communicating with each other, attenuating the possibility of friction.

Visual Rhetoric

One final implication that the applied research on emoji has produced is the fact that emoji are essentially visual rhetorical devices, rather than purely prefabricated informational pictograms, having evolved over a short period of time into rhetorical forms of persuasion in the classic sense (Aristotle 1952). As discussed throughout, emoji choices in a hybrid text carry great significance that surpasses any purported reinforcement of the written text or projection of nonverbal cues, and the like, onto the digital text. The same emoji may, in effect, be used to produce rhetorical effects at different levels. These are the product of the interplay of paradigmatic, syntagmatic, and associative structure. Consider a simple (albeit nontrivial) example – namely the smiley emoji (once again). What keeps the happy and sad emoji faces distinct (Figure 7.1)?

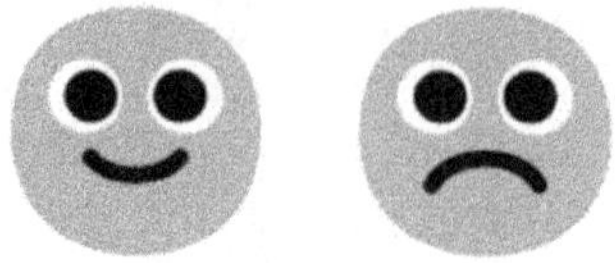

Figure 7.1 Happy versus sad emoji face

The answer is, needless to say, the orientation of the buccal outline, whereby in the happy face it slants upwards while in the sad face it slants downwards. While this may seem trivial, semiotically it is technically a signifier, the form of a sign that suggests a meaning, or signified (Saussure 1916). This same type of systematic contrastive cuing modality occurs across sign systems, which need not concern us here. Now, choosing one or the other emoji is a paradigmatic choice, because the selection is guided by the signifier–signified relation. This has a rhetorical substructure, however, since one or the other emoji would be placed in locations in a text where rhetorical effects such as agreement or disagreement, for example, are intended via the visual signifiers. The placement itself is guided by syntagmatic structure, which involves where the emoji are to be placed logically according to rhetorical sense. Finally, to complete the rhetorical effect, associative structure comes into play, whereby the selected and collocated emoji can be linked distributively so as to produce a commonality in meaning among what would otherwise be disparate concepts.

Emoji thus have the ability "to draw viewers into the argument's construction via the viewer's cognitive role in … filling in the unstated premise" (Blair 2004: 41). They are part of an ever-expanding visual rhetoric that, in an age of technology, can be utilized by anyone with a computer. Emoji thus produce multiple interpretations from the same specific image template (signifier–signified relation), so that what is unstated becomes expressed rhetorically.

Applications

The main aim of this book has been to assess how emoji are used, or can be used, in educational and healthcare settings as facilitators of communications and as activators or enhancers of learning. A concomitant objective has been to consider the supposed therapeutic effects of using emoji in clinical settings, including their overall ability to seemingly enhance well-being. The studies conducted in these areas (Chapters 2 and 4), together with the general literature on emoji, has allowed us concretely to make recommendations as to the significance of their utilization more broadly in education and healthcare.

Perhaps at no other time in the history of education and pedagogy in school contexts have teachers been so knowledgeable about what to do in the classroom or have so many sophisticated didactic tools at their disposal to help their students learn skills – from expertly designed textbooks to technologically sophisticated devices and online platforms for extending the classroom beyond its "four walls," as McLuhan (1960) had predicted decades ago (Chapter 6). In the era of the Internet, McLuhan's prognostication has certainly come about, as students and teachers interact not only within the confines of a traditional classroom but also beyond it through online media on a routine basis. Yet, despite the many strides that teachers and educators more generally have made over the years, and notwithstanding the many technological tools that they have at hand today, relatively few instructors have adopted the forms of our multimedia literacy world to help students achieve their potential with more facility and inclusivity, especially those who are struggling on account of various underprivileged or disadvantaged background reasons.

The underlying question that this type of investigation has raised is: Can the kinds of cognitive and expressive patterns involved in hybrid communications be transferred to the classroom or to healthcare communications to enhance learning and interactional fluidity? It was the little empirical research on addressing this question that led us to undertake several research projects that had implications for answering it to some extent. The main implications, and thus applications, of emoji use are summarized as follows. Overall, the incorporation of the students' emoji literacy into pedagogy allows teachers to take advantage of the cognitive shift that has occurred from the print age to the Internet age, which, in itself, promotes unconscious learning, given that students will much more easily understand novel content, such as the grammar, vocabulary, and lexicon involved in the language of academic literacy or in the symbolic structure of a discipline such as mathematics (especially in algebra and related branches). As discussed, emoji can even be employed as specific instructional techniques in teaching a foreign language. Applied emojistics, as we have termed it, like any applied discipline, is useful only insofar as it can provide concrete pedagogical insights, not overarching solutions or panaceas, that teachers can apply to their specific situations.

Healthcare

One of the central findings of the kind of research conducted and described here (Chapter 4), as well as can be gleaned from the general literature in this area, as sparse as it is, is that emoji facilitate healthcare communications in all kinds of situations. To cite Lai, Lee, and He (2021), with regard to clinician–patient digital interactions, emoji constitute a "powerful way for patients and doctors to communicate: The colorful symbols that are part of mainstream dialogue could provide patients a new way to be heard by their physicians."

As we also discussed, simple button terminals stationed around emergency departments featuring emoji reflecting a range of emotions are effective in monitoring doctor and patient sentiments in real time – a finding that has been extended to other areas of healthcare communications.

In a pertinent study, Lin and Luo (2023) found that by providing health information through hybrid forms of communication, with a salience on the visual modality, public health agencies can more effectively persuade people to adopt healthy behaviors, which is critical in the context of constantly emerging public health crises. The researchers examined how emoji shaped people's preventive and self-protective behaviors, finding that emoji attenuated the fear factor by injecting light-heartedness in a nonjudgmental way into the relevant communications. Overall, the relation between emoji literacy and health-related issues, from effective clinician–patient communications to the use of emoji in psychotherapy to enhance well-being, can be claimed to be a strong one. Among the features that define this relation, the following are worth highlighting here:

- *Emotional temperature.* Traditionally, practitioners gauge the emotional state of their patients by engaging with them in a face-to-face environment, asking questions, and assessing their body language. In digital communications, these aspects are transferred to the screen via emoji selections. Lu, Ai, Chen, Cao, and Mei (2022) developed a strategy that was designed to help people better monitor emotional well-being, which could also be used to better predict their behavior. Although their research was conducted in a different environment (the business workplace), the results are clearly transferable to the healthcare domain. The researchers monitored the use of emoji in online communications as a proxy for the emotions of interlocutors, enabling them to accurately predict their state of mind. Emoji thus allowed the researchers to take the "emotional temperature" of the interlocutors.
- *Emotional clues*. In a remote communication environment, it is difficult to pick up on the kind of emotional cues and signals that can be gleaned intuitively in a face-to-face setting. This is true even in video calls. As the previously mentioned study also found, these cues are intrinsic to emoji in a fundamental way, so that they are, ipso facto, conveyors of emotional cues, without any need to employ physical ones.
- *Reliable signs*. The study showed overall that emoji are reliable signs in conveying the emotional states of interlocutors. For instance, a smiley face was given more weight than a checkmark emoji. People who regularly used emoji to signify emotions tended to have better emotional health, regardless of whether the emoji they used were positive or negative.

In a similar study, Liu (2023) investigated whether emotional expressions and the types of emoji used are adjusted to digital contexts in accordance with facial displays. Over 1,200 Japanese participants were asked to select emoji in response to Internet chats so as to indicate the intensity of their responses. The results showed that, similar to facial displays, the participants expressed emotions through emoji more in positive contexts than in negative contexts, and more in private than in public contexts. They also tended to use euphemistic emoji in negative contexts to assuage a situation. As Linda Kaye (2018) has remarked, this area of research has documented that emoji are powerful devices for emotion and sentiment detection within textual discourse, thus constituting valuable signs for therapeutic purposes. Emoji have also been found to relate to a number of personality traits, such as emotional stability, extraversion, and agreeableness (Marengo, Giannotta, and Settanni 2017), suggesting they may have important functions for personality questionnaires in different domains of psychotherapy. This is particularly noteworthy given that openness is not always a dynamic in face-to-face first impressions.

The significant correlation between emoji and healthcare issues implies the need to consider systematically incorporating emoji into the education and healthcare spheres, as part of training students and practitioners in the new literacies. The Palangas study (Chapter 4), for instance, has clear implications for using such training systematically, since it showed that healthcare practitioners, in different disciplines and fields, came to understand the value of emoji communication gradually during the period of the course in which they had enrolled. Even those who were hesitant (for the reasons discussed) eventually came around to seeing the practicality of using emoji in all kinds of healthcare communicative contexts, especially since they realized that they did not destroy the politeness relation that they saw as crucial between doctor and patient (called a duality function). Focusing on how emoji communicate emotions and provide a mechanism for conveying empathy would be the central features of the relevant pedagogy.

In a pertinent study, Marzouk, He, and Lee (2022) found that the incorporation of emoji into traditionally word-only texts not only improved communication but also offered greater access to healthcare, "especially for vulnerable and marginalized populations with limited health literacy." The authors point out that health officials are now adding emoji to cardiopulmonary resuscitation guidelines and public health guidelines for handwashing, given that the research is so strongly suggestive of their effectiveness in getting the message across. As they conclude, in line with our own conclusions, given the ubiquity of new methods of communication and new literacies, practitioners must be exposed, formally, to new and effective modes of communicating health information to patients, despite the potential problems that this might involve. After all, problems emerge in any mode of discourse; emoji are no different in this regard.

Literacy in a Multimedia Age

The other primary goal of this book has been to investigate and discuss the role of emoji to determine whether developmental reading and writing students could demonstrate mastery of basic literacy skills via emoji use and how the same approach could benefit the teaching of literacy more generally in a multimedia age (Chapter 2). By incorporating the different literacies (verbal and nonverbal) into the classroom, the learning effects noted included the spontaneous crystallization of a semioliterate competence, that is, of the ability to navigate through the different literacies and to note the distinctive forms and functions of each one. In a nutshell, the Petcoff study showed that use of emoji constituted a transference mechanism that allowed students to project what they learned in the literacy classroom onto other areas of knowledge acquisition.

Analogous studies (Suleiman and Eltom 2019, Stavans, Eden, and Azar 2021) have examined the acquisition of academic literacy in a parallel way, finding as well that emoji facilitate its acquisition via their ability to induce students to link ideas between the verbal and visual modes of writing. As Semetsky (2019) has cogently argued, the activation of dormant semioliterate skills in students should be a primary goal of education, targeting them directly – as supported by the Petcoff pilot study. In both literacy training and psychotherapy, Semetsky defines semioliteracy as the discovery of meaning from different codes (verbal and nonverbal). As she states (2019): "In education, the dimension of meaning is often neglected, giving way as such to academic achievement." She sees edusemiotics, therefore, as a pivotal educational theory based on meaning creation and extraction via the different semiotic codes that we all utilize on a daily basis. Its main focus is, thus, the development of semioliteracy.

Semioliteracy training is a specific way to approach media literacy in general, which implies concrete knowledge of how the different media work and how they might be amalgamated to compose messages that may influence perspective and understanding. Traditional academic literacy is the process of extracting meaning from print and putting meaning into print. This process has traditionally been developed through formal schooling. However, there has always been a social power dynamic behind such literacy. Those with the highest levels tend, in fact, to be power brokers with the ability to make themselves heard and noticed. The evolving forms of new media literacies have emerged to attenuate this dynamic somewhat, even though academic literacy is still important for formal writing and learning situations. Emoji use in the classroom is a way to reach the levels required for such literacy, not to replace them.

Media literacy involves the influence of technological and global forces that have become intrinsic to everyday communication and literacy practices online. The ability to decipher, create, understand, and interpret digital texts has become essential to everyone. Without such broad semioliteracy today, people's ability to function in modern society diminishes considerably. Nonetheless, it is correct to say that there are two main literacies, an online and offline one, each one contextualized according to function. In schools, traditional literacy practices still prevail. However, as discussed here, online literacy can be incorporated in the classroom to allow students the choice to move back and forth between the literacies.

Weigle and Caprino (2018) discuss caveats that emoji use may present, such as the "potential for some students to create unrealistic or stereotypical representations of characters, classmates, or themselves." However, such occasions actually can be turned to advantage practically, since they can be used to encourage discussions around digital citizenship and inclusivity. As Sexton and Beegle (2020) observe, above all else, the modern classroom is where students encounter academic literacy likely for the first time. To make them realize that academic language is critical to school achievement, and foundational for the comprehension of content-rich subjects, the mechanism of emoji-based instruction can be used to move over to such language in a way that is itself "meaning-rich" and "omnipresent in students' everyday lives." Therefore, "it behooves educators to explore ways to make emoji work more productively in teaching this critical foundational skill."

Inclusivity

One of the social aspects of emoji use is its propensity to eliminate stigmas involved in the perception of literacy acquisition, given that emoji use is inclusive, no matter the background or predispositions of students. Unlike the perceptions evoked by the word choices and utterance styles of academic literacy, which vary from positive to highly stigmatic (when used improperly), emoji are part of a common visual language that bears no inbuilt register- or literacy-based judgments. By their typically cartoonish nature, they assure students, patients, and virtually everyone else who is on digital writing media that one does not need to be literate at the highest levels to get a message across. Moreover, as discussed throughout this book, emoji can actually help people express themselves in ways that words often cannot and, indirectly, allow the voices of those who have, traditionally, been underserved and even ignored to be heard equitably.

Of course, dangers of miscommunication (not to mention bias and prejudice) can creep into emoji use. But the fact that this can be detected by virtually anyone who is emoji literate indicates that there is an inbuilt detection system at the level of the emoji interpretant. To reiterate here, an emoji, such as the angel 😇 emoji, will convey meanings that are accrued in cultural settings. So, in most western cultures, it stands for innocence or a good deed, among other related meanings. However, it is a sign of bereavement in China, where it could also be perceived as a threat. Moreover, emoji can evoke different interpretations depending on the generation of users. So, while there are impediments to inclusivity in emoji use, by and large, they bespeak of phatic communion, no matter the background of the user.

Education

A primary value of emoji in education is that they make the classroom relevant, since they are already a big part of how we communicate in our digital world today. As such, they can be used as a metalanguage for imparting knowledge, like any pedagogical metalanguage, as discussed in Chapter 6, and thus used to introduce and explain concepts in, say, a foreign language, mathematics, history, and so on. Moreover, they are unmarked for age and level of achievement, since students of all ages and levels use them, and thus can be adapted accordingly (Teixera 2022). This is not to make emoji the primary literacy, but rather to employ it creatively to teach the broader academic literacy and to help impart novel ideas in all kinds of disciplines in a synchronous way with existing social patterns of communication outside of the classroom. As such, emoji bear concrete implications for activating learning processes in a bimodal way, activating R-Mode processes and L-Mode processes in tandem – that is to say, they have the ability to produce image schemas in the mind (R-Mode thinking) that become the basis for abstractions of various kinds related to specific disciplines (L-Mode thinking). This makes emoji potentially highly useful as a means for enhancing learning generally. From our own studies and the ever-increasing literature on emoji in education, the following five (putative) acquisitional properties of emoji use can be highlighted for the sake of argument:

(1) Emoji add visuality to the teaching-learning process, an R-Mode process, making the emoji metalanguage especially useful in the early or initial stages of novel learning.
(2) They attract and retain the attention of learners, who become involved in some learning task via a visual presentation (again an R-Mode function).
(3) They encourage learners to concretely demonstrate what they have learned with digital media, which immerses them into the cognitive space that learning entails and, in turn, allows them to unconsciously transfer such learning to other areas (an R-Mode to L-Mode shift).
(4) They can be selected adaptively to specific learners, because they present concepts, including complex ones, in ways that are understandable across styles.

(5) They make the classroom more interactive and inclusive, as discussed several times.

The effectiveness of emoji-based (and other multimedia) techniques has been corroborated by extensive research that has shown, in a nutshell, that retention and recall of information is significantly improved when the senses are engaged in absorbing it. For example, a study by Rasul, Bukhsh, and Batool in 2011 found that students experienced visual teaching techniques as playing an important role in their learning levels. Kurniawan (2016: 180) studied the connection between visual teaching and the enhancement of speaking skills, including pronunciation, finding a significant correlation between the two. The likely reason for such findings is that the processing of visual information is not confined to a single region of the brain, although specific areas in the right hemisphere are activated in processing visual input (R-Mode learning). Rather, different neural modules are involved in helping the brain process novel input. So, emoji carry information that is converted by the brain into neuronal activities that are conducive to the effective processing of new input (Yuasa, Saito, and Mukawa 2011). The brain first processes the meanings of emoji holistically, subsequently extracting the abstract relations in them, in a connected or distributed fashion (as general research on visuality has shown, such as Hickok, Bellugi, and Klima 2001). There is a general caveat, however, with regard to emoji pedagogy, which must be emphasized repeatedly – namely, the problem of culture-based interpretation: Which image is the appropriate one culturally? So, when teaching visually, one must keep in mind the interpretive function of images – what may appear neutral to some cultures may be perceived negatively in others.

A key aspect of emoji-based learning is that it activates the R-Mode, which involves intuitive thinking, and is the likely source for getting students to more easily acquire the structures present in novel input in a spontaneous way. The learning unit then becomes assimilated, activating L-Mode mechanisms, again spontaneously, which involve organizational thinking, allowing students to formalize their acquired knowledge. This is consistent with the psychological research on mental development more broadly, such as Jean Piaget's classic research, as mentioned previously (Piaget 1969). Piaget showed, in a phrase, that children progress from a sensory and concrete stage of mind (R-Mode learning) to a reflective and abstract one (L-Mode thinking). Around the age of two, children, according to Piaget's observations, start to develop symbolic abilities derived from mental images. As these become more dynamic, they prepare the child for more abstract thinking. In terms of emoji-based teaching, the developmental stages documented by Piaget can be formulated in terms of the flow of learning that starts via the R-Mode, corresponding to both the sensory-motor and concrete operational stages (to varying degrees), and ends in the L-Mode formal-logical thinking stage.

Emoji Pedagogy

English instructor Lindsay Clandfield (2017) is one of a growing number of teachers who utilize emoji as pedagogical devices systematically, so as to activate the learning processes described here in their classrooms. Such ever-expanding pedagogical practices cumulatively support the findings of our own projects and the general literature on the psychology of emoji use. What stands out is how easily emoji can be applied to the teaching of specific skills, not only literacy-based ones. For example, Clandfield suggests using emoji as writing prompts, whereby students are asked to create, say, a paragraph that includes them. Illustrative prompts include the following:

> Last night I had the strangest dream …
>
> 
>
> It was eight o'clock and the dinner party was almost ready …
>
> 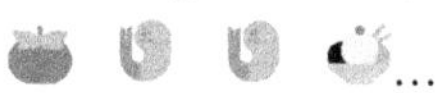
>
> I come from a very interesting family …
>
> 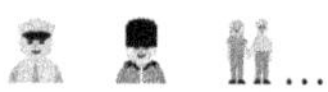

A perusal of similar pedagogical articles and projects leads us to underscore a few general ideas that emerge from the implementation of different approaches to emoji pedagogy:

- Emoji-based techniques are versatile creative devices alongside other kinds of techniques. Each use is initially an R-Mode stimulator, since it presents information in a compact and understandable way that is part of how students now write. They activate the learning flow, to varying degrees. After this is set in motion, emoji immerse students into the subject matter in various ways according to discipline, thus activating L-Mode reflection.
- Emoji-based activities should be given the same treatment and weight as other techniques, as the Petcoff study showed; otherwise, the students will tend not to take them seriously in the long run.
- Both teachers and students must find emoji use enjoyable; otherwise, it might become counterproductive.
- Advanced students who are in firm control of the required L-Mode skills through previous training will not have to spend as much time on the use of emoji to activate bimodal learning. When students have mastered the L-Mode aspects of a concept, then they will be in a position to integrate them with the R-Mode ones as they perform other tasks in the classroom.

On the motivational front, emoji pedagogy seems to favor several learning processes that can be summarized as follows:

(1) *A sense of play.* Emoji tend to impart a sense that learning new concepts is an enjoyable process, much like playing with symbols in a ludic way.
(2) *Improvisation.* Emoji present concrete opportunities for improvisation, as discussed several times.
(3) *Simulation.* They simulate content derived from real-world experiences, turning it into small-scale models of those experiences.
(4) *Amalgamation.* This involves knowing how to extract, use, remix, and amalgamate different emoji within the context of a specific learning task.
(5) *Multiple perspectives.* Emoji pedagogy involves utilizing multiple perspectives made possible by multimedia communication, so that bimodal processes can be activated spontaneously.

AI and Emoji

In a world where AI is spreading throughout society, taking over many of the tasks that were done, literally, by hand, it comes as little surprise to find that research on emoji in the framework of AI is now a target area within cognitive science. As Piriyatamwong (2022) has pointed out, emoji-based research now covers a broad range, from predicting what the appropriate emoji should be in a specific location within a text, via Natural Language Processing algorithms, to providing simulative test models of how the semiotic and discursive functions of emoji may unfold in the brain. The machine does not understand what each emoji means, unlike humans. But it is good at executing things as per specific instructions, like checking on patterns of usage. Piriyatamwong gives several illustrative examples. For example, the fire emoji 🔥 is now a basic one in everyday communications, explained by Unicode as indicating fire itself, flames, certain manufactured tools, and so on. Now, as Piriyatamwong (2022) notes, "when we type 'lit,' the emoji '🔥' also shows up although 'lit' is not a keyword associated with '🔥' in the Unicode database." Instead, the power of the AI lies in its ability to infer that it is connected to the emoji. This has clear implications for studying how signs and texts are interpreted in the human brain vicariously (Neuman, Danesi, and Vilenchik 2023). What such research implies is that "When we learn something, the brain propagates the just-learned knowledge through its neural network, keeping the knowledge in memory, and reusing it later when triggered," which is consistent with bimodality theory. As Piriyatamwong (2022) concludes:

> The process called the pre-processing step first turns the input text ("knowledge") into individual words and emojis (known as "tokens") and assigns them numerical labels to be understood by the neural network. A "probability" is assigned to each and every

emoji, and the one with the highest chance is picked. But how are these probabilities calculated? This is the neural network's work. Basically, it does a lot of mathematical computations, from the first randomly-assigned probabilities, then where the neural is connected or joined, it does some addition, multiplication, or scaling to "update" the probabilities for each emoji again.

An area of AI-based investigation that is highly significant is detecting "hatemoji" on the Internet, or emoji that are twisted in nefarious hateful ways. A research team at the Oxford Internet Institute (Kirk, Vidgen, Röttger, and Hale 2021) found that online posts that contain hate speech are actually difficult to detect because of the hatemoji themselves. For example, algorithms have a hard time evaluating the monkey emoji as potentially a hatemoji, because it is rarely used in this way in the majority of posts. Because of this problem, the Oxford team developed a database of around 4,000 sentences that contained different hatemoji. They then used it to train an AI model in the usual way. The AI-based model was then tested in the use of hate speech online against minorities, different gender-identified communities, and the like. The model increased detection efficiency considerably. Needless to say, using this AI, which has been made publicly available, will be a useful resource for educational reasons, since it can inform the teacher as to what to avoid, as well as providing context for discussing inclusivity in the classroom.

Epilogue

The objective of this book has been to discuss, illustrate, and present data and arguments for incorporating emoji into educational and healthcare communication settings. These are actually the two sides of the same coin, so to speak, since they both involve reaching people (learners or patients) via a form of contemporary communication – emoji – that is highly understandable and inclusive. The supportive studies and projects discussed in this book can be said to constitute the groundwork for developing an "applied emojistics," intended to examine emoji applications to areas that have practical and important relevance to society (such as healthcare and education). Much like applied linguistics, which at first concerned itself with the application of theoretical linguistics to language teaching practices but has since been expanded to include broader applications to real-life needs (including speech therapy, language policies, etc.), applied emojistics has, in our view, concrete implications for real-life needs as well.

The Oxford Dictionary was right after all in 2015, choosing an emoji for its word of the year, sensing that emoji had captured a crossroads moment in time. The question of how emoji will evolve is a McLuhanian one, given that it involves understanding the relation between social evolution and technological change. At present, emoji are part and parcel of everyday interactions and have even made their way into the field of AI, as mentioned earlier. Already in 2017, the MIT Media Lab produced DeepMoji, a deep neural network algorithm for sentiment analysis trained on more than a billion emoji occurrences on Twitter, outperforming human subjects in detecting sarcasm and other variable interpretive modes in emoji usage. Deep learning algorithms are now used to understand the flow of a message and can suggest what emoji are appropriate as the message unfolds, constituting an expanding N-gram analysis (algorithmic analysis that predict sequences in speech and symbol systems) that includes emoji.

The routine use of emoji has many social implications, as discussed throughout this book. It signals, above all else, a paradigm shift away from print literacy as the central form of writing to a broader multimedia blending of literacies. Emoji have come forth to effectively signal that the traditional distinction no longer exists between separate verbal and visual modes of representation and communication. It remains to be seen what uses, if any, emoji will have in the future as communications technologies advance, given that emoji themselves were made available by a certain novel technology. As McLuhan (1969: 5) wrote with regard to electronic writing even before the advent of emoji: "We live invested in an electric information environment that is quite as imperceptible to us as water is to fish." The kinds of signs and sign systems that will emerge in the ever-expanding "Technosphere" will affect how we communicate and even think in the future.

Unlike the print age, which spread after the invention of the printing press and imposed the use of the written word in most forms of communication and knowledge-making, the current Internet age encourages various modes of writing in tandem with script. Adopting the hybrid mode (words and emoji) for informal interactions has become more of a necessity than an option for most people, and so, incorporating it into areas of concern is now a necessity as well. That said, there are several provisos that are relevant to emphasize one more time, by way of conclusion. First, not all forms of writing are hybrid, especially in areas such as academia, science, journalism, lawmaking, and the like; emoji are constrained to communication in contexts that involve the informal register, used largely to impart a friendly and positive tone to messages. Second, emoji writing depends on technology, with emoji characters just a click away (so to speak); without this easy accessibility, it is unlikely that emoji would have spread so broadly in the first place. Emoji allow for an easy way to add a whole array of meanings (summarized in this chapter) that are not always possible to realize so easily with verbal forms. Third, the rise of emoji is historically based. That is, they would not have spread if the modern mind was not conditioned to accept visuality in daily communications as a natural outgrowth of various other trends. One of these, as mentioned several times, is the comic book, which blends images and words in a narrative framework. Early twentieth-century art movements such as Dada and Futurism also showed that the printed word, laid out in a linear fashion, might have run its course as a means to encode meanings about a broadening technological world.

The advent of digital technology simply provided the physical tools to make new forms of writing, blending the verbal and visual, a matter of routine. As *The Matrix* (1999) emphasized, the digital age has reshaped our consciousness. Like the protagonist of that movie, Neo, we now live "on" and "through" the computer screen. Our engagement with reality is largely shaped by that screen, whose technical name is the *matrix*, defined as the network of circuits that constitute a computer screen. But the same word also meant "womb" in Latin. The movie's transparent subtext was that, with the advent of the computer era, people are born through two kinds of wombs – the biological and the technological. The appearance and spread of emoji could only have occurred in the matrix in which we all live. As a consequence, the way we read and write messages on a screen, and conceptualize them, is different than how we used to write them on paper. Of course, visual images in the form of illustrations were always a possibility, but a difficult one to carry out. With digital keyboards and apps now making emoji easily available, the semiotic and discursive function of images has become part and parcel of how we communicate and think. Ignoring this fact in areas such as healthcare and education would be anachronistic and unwise, as argued throughout this book.

We end with the words of Dr. Shuhan He, who was one of our interviewees for this book, a prominent physician and medical researcher who has become a leading voice in the promotion of emoji literacy in the healthcare area. His words encapsulate the overall theme and objective of this book (cited in *Newswise*, www.newswise.com/articles/emoji):

> The need to listen to patients is at the core of our mission as physicians, and the use of emoji is a great opportunity to take communication to another level. It's tempting to dismiss emoji as a millennial fad, but they possess the power of standardization, universality and familiarity, and in the hands of physicians and other health care providers could represent a new and highly effective way to communicate pictorially with patients … It's clear that emoji have become part of the global, mainstream conversation, and that medical societies and physician committees and organizations need to take them seriously.

References

Adams, F. (1849). *The Genuine Works of Hippocrates*. London: Sydenham Society.

Agarwal, A. K., Hahn, L., Petullo, A., Rosin, R., and Merchant, R. M. (2020). Capturing Real-Time Emergency Department Sentiment: A Feasibility Study Using Touch-Button Terminals. *Annals of Emergency Medicine* 75(6): 727–732.

Albright, J., and Luke, A. (2012). *Pierre Bourdieu and Literacy Education*. London: Routledge.

Alexander, K. E., Ogle, T., Hoberg, H., Linley, L., and Bradford, N. (2021). Patient Preferences for Using Technology in Communication about Symptoms Post Hospital Discharge. *Biomedical Central Health Service Research* 21: 141. https://doi.org/10.1186/s12913-021-06119-7.

Allen, K. et al. (2017). How I Feel about My School: The Construction and Validation of a Measure of Wellbeing at School for Primary School Children. *Clinical Child Psychology and Psychiatry* 23(1): 25–41.

Alshenqeeti, H. (2016). Are Emojis Creating a New or Old Visual Language for New Generations? A Socio-semiotic Study. *Advances in Language and Literary Studies* 7. https://ssrn.com/abstract=3709343.

Amit, E., Danziger, S., and Smith, P. K. (2022). Medium Is a Powerful Message: Pictures Signal Less Power than Words. *Organizational Behavior and Human Decision Processes* 169. https://doi.org/10.1016/j.obhdp.2022.104132.

An, J., Zhang, P., Li, T., and Teng, Y. (2018). Factors Influencing Emoji Usage in Smartphone Mediated Communications. In G. Chowdhury, J. McLeod, V. Gillet, and P. Willett (eds.), *Transforming Digital Worlds: iConference 2018: Lecture Notes in Computer Science*, vol. 10766, 423–428. Cham: Springer. https://doi.org/10.1007/978-3-319-78105-1_46.

Andel, S. A., de Vreede, T., Spector, P. E., et al. (2020). Do Social Features Help in Video-Centric Online Learning Platforms? A Presence Perspective. *Computers in Human Behavior* 113: 106505. https://doi.org/10.1016/j.chb.2020.106505.

Angotti, R., and Bayo, I. (2012). Making Kinections: Using Video Game Technology to Teach Math. *Prato CIRN Community Informatics Conference*: 1–6.

Arendale, D. R. (2014). History of Learning Assistance in U.S. Postsecondary Education. In H. R. Boylan and B. S. Bonham (eds.), *Developmental Education: Readings on Its Past, Present, and Future*, 28–57. New York: St. Martin's.

Aristotle. (1952). *Rhetoric*. In W. D. Ross (ed.), *The Works of Aristotle*, vol. 11. Oxford: Clarendon Press.

Arnheim, R. (1969). *Visual Thinking*. Berkeley: University of California Press.

Assadi, R., Lotfinejad, N., Ziae, A., and Ganjali, B. (2020). Medical Emoji for Clinical Signs and Symptoms: A Comprehensive Qualitative Study. medRxiv. https://doi.org/10.1101/2020.11.28.20240085.

Baer, E. (1988). *Medical Semiotics*. New York: University Press of America.

Bai, Q., Dan, Q., Mu, Z., and Yang, M. (2019). A Systematic Review of Emoji: Current Research and Future Perspectives. *Frontiers in Psychology* 15. https://doi.org/10.3389/fpsyg.2019.02221.

Bakhtin, M. M. (1981). *The Dialogic Imagination: Four Essays*. Austin: University of Texas Press.

Barden, O. (2012). If We Were Cavemen We'd Be Fine: Facebook as a Catalyst for Critical Literacy Learning by Dyslexic Sixth-Form Students. *Literacy* 46: 123–132.

Bargh, J. A., and Chartrand, T. L. (2000). Studying the Mind in the Middle: A Practical Guide to Priming and Automaticity Research:23–36. In H. Reis and C. Judd (eds.), *Handbook of Research Methods in Social Psychology*. New York: Cambridge University Press.

Barinaga-López, B., Puente-Bienvenido, H., and Newball, A. (2022). A Systematic Review of Trends and Gaps in the Production of Scientific Knowledge on the Sociopolitical Impacts of Emojis in Computer-Mediated Communication. *Cogent Social Sciences* 8(1). http://doi.org/10.1080/23311886.2022.2151096.

Barnum, J. F. (1993). Medical Diagnosis through Semiotics: Giving Meaning to the Sign. *Annals of Internal Medicine* 119: 939–943.

Barthes, R. (1964). Rhetoric of the Image. In C. Handa (ed.), *Visual Rhetoric in a Visual World: A Critical Sourcebook*. New York: Bedford/St. Martin's.

Barthes, R. (1977). *Image-Music-Text*. London: Fontana.

Barthes, R. (1981). *Camera Lucida*. New York: Hill and Wang.

Baudrillard, J. (1983). *Simulations*. New York: Semiotexte.

Beißwenger, M., and Pappert, S. (2019). How to Be Polite with Emojis: A Pragmatic Analysis of Face Work Strategies in an Online Learning Environment. *European Journal of Applied Linguistics* 7: 225–254.

Benavides-Vanegas, F. S. (2020). Emoticons, Memes and Cyberbullying: Gender Equality in Colombia. *Social Semiotics* 30: 328–343.

Berard, B. (2018). I Second that Emoji: The Standards, Structures, and Social Production of Emoji. *First Monday* 32(9). https://doi.org/10.5210/fm.v23i9.9381.

Bhattacharya, S., Singh, A., and Marzo, R. R. (2019). Delivering Emoji/Icon-Based Universal Health Education Messages through Smartphones. *AIMS Public Health* 6(3): 242–247.

Bivins, R. (2007). "The English Disease" or "Asian Rickets"? Medical Responses to Postcolonial Immigration. *Bulletin of the History of Medicine* 81: 533–568.

Black, R. W. (2008). Just Don't Call Them Cartoons: The New Literacy Spaces of Anime, Manga and Fanfiction. In J. Coiro, M. Knobel, C. Lankshear, and D. Leu (eds.), *Handbook of Research on New Literacies*, 538–610. New York: Lawrence Erlbaum Associates.

Blair, J. A. (2004). The Rhetoric of Visual Arguments. In C. A. Hill and M. Helmers (eds.), *Defining Visual Rhetorics*, 41–61. Mahwah, NJ: Lawrence Erlbaum Associates.

Borgman, J., and McArdle, C. (2019). *Personal, Accessible, Responsive, Strategic: Resources and Strategies for Online Writing Instructors*. Denver: University Press of Colorado.

Bourdieu, P. (1972). *Outline of a Theory of Practice*. Cambridge: Cambridge University Press.

Braun, V., and Clarke, V. (2012). Thematic Analysis. In H. Cooper, P. M. Camic, D. L. Long et al. (eds.), *Research Designs: Quantitative, Qualitative, Neuropsychological, and Biological*, 57–71. American Psychological Association. https://doi.org/10.1037/13620-004.

Brown, N. (2022). Emoji Are Shown to Be as Effective as Numerical Pain Scales in Judging Patient Pain Levels in the Hospital. *Medical Xpress*. https://medicalxpress.com/news/2022-07-emoji-shown-effective-numerical-pain.html.

Bryden, J., Funk, S., and Jansen, V. (2013). Word Usage Mirrors Community Structure in the Online Social Network Twitter. *EPJ Data Science* 2: 3. www.epjdatascience.com/content/2/1/3.

Burnum, J. F. (1993). Medical Diagnosis through Semiotics: Giving Meaning to the Sign. *Annals of Internal Medicine* 119: 939–943.

Butterworth, S. E., Giuliano, T. A., White, J., Cantu, L., and Fraser, K. C. (2019). Sender Gender Influences Emoji Interpretation in Text Messages. *Frontiers in Psychology* 10. https://doi.org/10.3389/fpsyg.2019.00784.

Callender, J., Bridge, P., Al-Samarraie, F., and Blair, D. (2022). The Use of Emoji to Establish Student Wellbeing: Does the Image Reflect the Reality? *Journal of Radiotherapy in Practice* 22: e30. https://doi.org/10.1017/S1460396921000704.

Carr, N. (2011). *The Shallows: What The Internet Is Doing to Our Brains*. New York: Norton.

Carr, N. (2015). *The Glass Cage: How Our Computers Are Changing Us*. New York: Norton.

Carroll, L. (1865). *Alice's Adventures in Wonderland*. London: Macmillan.

Chadwick, J., and Mann, W. N. (1950). *The Medical Works of Hippocrates*. Oxford: Blackwell.

Chatzichristos, C., Morante, M., Andreadis, N., et al. (2020). Emojis Influence Autobiographical Memory Retrieval from Reading Words: An fMRI-based Study. *PLoS One* 15(7): e0234104. https://doi.org/10.1371/journal.pone.0234104.

Chen, B. (2023). Emojis Aid Social Media Sentiment Analysis: Stop Cleaning Them Out! *Medium*. https://towardsdatascience.com/emojis-aid-social-media-sentiment-analysis-stop-cleaning-them-out-bb32a1e5fc8e.

Cheng, L., Yuxiu, S., and Li, J. (2020). Aggressiveness of Emojis Before the Court: A Sociosemiotic Interpretation. *Social Semiotics* 30: 365–378.

Christofalos, A. L., Feldman, L. B., and Sheridan, H. (2020). Semantic Congruency Facilitates Memory for Emojis. *Proceedings of the Fifth International Workshop on Emoji Understanding and Applications in Social Media*, 63–68. Association for Computational Linguistics.

Churches, O., Nicholls, M., Thiessen, M., Kohler, M., and Keage, H. (2014). Emoticons in Mind: An Event-Related Potential Study. *Social Neuroscience* 9: 196–202.

Clandfield, L. (2017). Emoji Lesson Pack. *Cambridge: Technology and Digital*. www.cambridge.org/elt/blog/2017/06/08/5_ways_teachers_use_emoji/.

Clay, M. (1966). *Reading: The Patterning of Complex Behaviour*. Auckland: Heinemann.

Clough, S., Morrow, E., Mutlu, B., Turkstra, L., and Duff, M. C. (2023). Emotion Recognition of Faces and Emoji in Individuals with Moderate–Severe Traumatic Brain Injury. *Brain Injury* 37(7): 596–610. http://doi.org/10.1080/02699052.2023.2181401.

Cohn, N., Engelen, J., and Schilperoord, J. (2019). The Grammar of Emoji? Constraints on Communicative Pictorial Sequencing. *Cognitive Research* 4(33). https://doi.org/10.1186/s41235-019-0177-0.

Cohn, N., Roijackers, T., Schaap, R., and Engelen, J. (2018). Are Emoji a Poor Substitute for Words? Sentence Processing with Emoji Substitutions. *Proceedings of the 40th Annual Conference of the Cognitive Science Society*, 1524–1529. The Cognitive Science Society. http://mindmodeling.org/cogsci2018/papers/0295/0295.pdf.

Conway, M. A. (2009). Episodic Memories. *Neuropsychologia* 47(11): 2305–2313.

Correa, S. (2021). How Emojis Have Changed the Way We Communicate. www.makeuseof.com/how-emojis-have-changed-the-way-we-communicate/.

Crombie, P. (2020). Faces, Hearts and Thumbs: Exploring the Use of Emoji in Online Teacher–Student Communications in Higher Education. *Journal of Academic Language and Learning* 14(1): 30–41.

Crystal, D. (2011). *Internet Linguistics: A Student Guide*. New York: Routledge.

Csíkszentmihályi, M. (1990). *Flow: The Psychology of Optimal Experience*. London: Harper and Row.

Dainas, A., and Herring, S. (2021). Interpreting Emoji Pragmatics. In C. Xie, F. Yus, and H. Haberland (eds.), *Approaches to Internet Pragmatics: Theory and Practice*, 107–144. Amsterdam: John Benjamins.

Damasio, A. R. (1994). *Descartes' Error: Emotion, Reason, and the Human Brain*. New York: G. P. Putnam.

Danesi, M. (1986). Research on the Brain's Hemispheric Functions: Implications for Second Language Pedagogy. *Lenguas Modernas* 18: 99–113.

Danesi, M. (2003). *Second Language Teaching: A View from the Right Side of the Brain*. Dordrecht: Kluwer.

Danesi, M. (2015). *Il cervello in aula: Neurolingistica e didattica delle lingue*. Perugia: Guerra.

Danesi, M. (2016). *The Semiotics of Emoji*. London: Bloomsbury.

Danesi, M. (2017). *Language and Mathematics: An Interdisciplinary Guide*. Berlin: Mouton de Gruyter.

Danesi, M. (2022). Emotional Wellbeing and the Semiotic Translation of Emojis. In S. Petrilli and M. Ji (eds.), *Exploring the Translatability of Emotions: Cross-Cultural and Transdisciplinary Encounters*, 323–344. Cham: Palgrave.

Dangor, J. (2017). Mayo Clinic Study Finds Emojis Promising Tool for Tracking Cancer Patients' Quality of Life. *Mayo Clinic*. https://newsnetwork.mayoclinic.org/discussion/physical-activity-data-emojis-on-apple-watch-correlated-with-patient-reported-outcomes/.

Davies, J. (2012). Facework on Facebook as a New Literacy Practice. *Computers & Education* 59: 19–29.

Davies, J., McKenna, M., Denner, K., Bayley, J., and Morgan, M. (2022). The Emoji Current Mood and Experience Scale: The Development and Initial Validation of an Ultra-Brief, Literacy Independent Measure of Psychological Health. *Journal of Mental Health*. https://doi.org/10.1080/09638237.2022.2069694.

Davis, D. S. (2021). Literacy Instruction and Social Justice: Disciplinary Literacy as a Tool for Disrupting Inequities. *SRATE Journal* 30(2).

Deely, J. (2001). *Four Ages of Understanding: The First Postmodern Survey of Philosophy from Ancient Times to the Turn of the Twentieth Century*. Toronto: University of Toronto Press.

Dewey, J. (1902). *The Child and the Curriculum*. Chicago: University of Chicago Press.

Dewey, J. (1916). *Democracy and Education*. New York: Macmillan.

Dhawan, C. (2021). *Digital Body Language: How to Build Trust and Connection, No Matter the Distance*. New York: St. Martin's Press.

Doiron, J. G. (2018). Emojis: Visual Communication in Higher Education. *International Journal of Teaching, Education and Learning* 2(2): 1–11.

Donga, M. (2019). Educatief spel met emoji-taal: Wat voel ik? *Onderwijs van Morgen*. www.onderwijsvanmorgen.nl/educatief-spel-met-emoji-taal-wat-voel-ik/.

Eco, U. (1974). *A Theory of Semiotics*. Bloomington: Indiana University Press.

Eco, U. (1979). *The Role of the Reader. Explorations in the Semiotics of Texts*. Bloomington: Indiana University Press.

Eco, U. (2010). Aristotle, Poetics and Rhetoric. In T. A. Sebeok and M. Danesi (eds.), *Encyclopedic Dictionary of Semiotics*, 57–58. Berlin: Mouton de Gruyter.

Ede, L., and Lunsford, A. A. (2009). Among the Audience: On Audience in an Age of New Literacies. In M. E. Weiser, B. M. Fehler, and A. M. Gonzalez (eds.), *Engaging Audience: Writing in an Age of New Literacies*, 42–72. Urbana, IL: National Council of Teachers of English.

Edwards, J. (2009). *Language and Identity*. Cambridge: Cambridge University Press.

Efron, D. (1941). *Gesture, Race, and Culture*. The Hague: Mouton.

Ekman, P. (1985). *Telling Lies*. New York: Norton.

Ekman, P. (1989). The Argument and Evidence about Universals in Facial Expressions of Emotion. In H. Wagner and A. Manstead (eds.), *Handbook of Social Psychophysiology*, 143–164. Chichester: Wiley.

Ekman, P. (2003). *Emotions Revealed*. New York: Holt.

Ekman, P., and Friesen, W. V. (1971). Constants across Cultures in the Face and Emotion. *Journal of Personality and Social Psychology* 17: 124–129.

Emanuel, E. J., and Emanuel, L. L. (1992). Four Models of the Physician–Patient Relationship. *Journal of the American Medical Association* 267(16): 2221–2226.

Evans, V. (2017). *The Emoji Code: The Linguistics Behind Smiley Faces and Scaredy Cats*. New York: Picador.

Fallows, R. R., and Hilsabeck, R. C. (2012). Visual Puzzles in a Mixed Clinical Sample. *The Clinical Neuropsychologist* 26: 942–950.

Fane, J. (2017). Using Emoji as a Tool to Support Child Wellbeing from a Strengths-Based Approach. *Learning Communities: International Journal of Learning in Social Contexts* 21: 96–107.

Fane, J., MacDougall, C., Jovanovic, J., Redmond, G., and Gibbs, L. (2018). Exploring the Use of Emoji as a Visual Research Method for Eliciting Young Children's Voices in Childhood Research. *Early Child Development and Care* 188(3): 359–374.

Farifteh, S., Mohammadi-Aria, A., Kiamanesh, A., and Mofid, B. (2014). The Impact of Laughter Yoga on the Stress of Cancer Patients Before Chemotherapy. *Iran Journal of Cancer Prevention* 7(4): 179–183.

Fauconnier, G., and Turner, M. (2002). *The Way We Think: Conceptual Blending and the Mind's Hidden Complexities*. New York: Basic.

Ferré, P., Haro, J., Pérez-Sánchez, M., Moreno, I., and Hinojosa, J. A. (2022). Emoji-SP, the Spanish Emoji Database: Visual Complexity, Familiarity, Frequency of Use, Clarity, and Emotional Valence and Arousal Norms for 1031 Emojis. *Behavior Research Methods* 55: 1715–1733. https://doi.org/10.3758/s13428-022-01893-6.

Foster, C. (2018). Why I Let My Students Use Emojis in Writing Assignments. *We Are Teachers*. www.weareteachers.com/teaching-with-emojis/.

Foucault, M. (1972). *The Archeology of Knowledge*. A. M. Sheridan Smith (trans.). New York: Pantheon.

Freedman, A. (2014). View of Cultural Literacy in the Empire of Emoji Signs: Who Is Crying with Joy? *First Monday* 23(9). https://doi.org/10.5210/fm.v23i9.9395.

Freire, P. (1970). *Pedagogy of the Oppressed*. New York: Continuum.

Frensch, P. A., and Runger, D. (2003). Implicit learning. *Current Directions in Psychological Science* 12: 13–18.

Freud, S. (1901). *The Interpretation of Dreams*. New York: Avon.

Gallagher, J. R., and Avgoustopoulos, R. E. (2023): Emojination Facilitates Inclusive Emoji Design Through Technical Writing: Fitting Tactical Technical Communication Inside Institutional Structures. *Journal of Technical Writing and Communication* 54(1): 93–112. https://doi.org/10.25384/SAGE.c.6460845.v1.

Gardner, M. (1998). A Quarter Century of Recreational Mathematics. *Scientific American* 279: 68–75.

Ge-Stadnyk, J., and Gretzel, U. (2018). Emoji Rhetoric: A Social Media Influencer Perspective. *Journal of Marketing Management* 34(2):1–24.

Gee, J. P. (1989). What Is Literacy? *Journal of Education* 1: 18–25.

Gee, J. P. (1996). *Social Linguistics and Literacies: Ideology in Discourses*. London: Taylor & Francis.

Gee, J. P. (2003). *What Video Games Have to Teach Us*. New York: St. Martin's.

Gee, J. P. (2015). *The New Literacy Studies*. New York: Routledge.

Gibson, W., Huang, P., and Yu, Q. (2018). Emoji and Communicative Action: The Semiotics, Sequence and Gestural Actions of "Face Covering Hand." *Discourse, Context & Media* 26: 91–99.

Gilster, P. (1998). *Digital Literacy*. New York: John Wiley.

Glass, A. L., and Kang, M. (2018). Dividing Attention in the Classroom Reduces Exam Performance. *Educational Psychology* 39(3): 395–408.

Glikson, E., Cheshin, A., and Van Kleef, G. A. (2018). The Dark Side of a Smiley: Effects of Smiling Emoticons on Virtual First Impressions. *Social Psychological and Personality Science* 9: 614–625.

Goffman, E. (1959). *The Presentation of Self in Everyday Life*. Garden City, NJ: Doubleday.

Goffman, E. (1963). *Behavior in Public Places*. New York: Free Press.

Goffman, E. (1974). *Frame Analysis*. New York: Harper and Row.

Goffman, E. (1978). Response Cries. *Language* 54: 787–815.

Goldberg, E., and Costa, L. D. (1981). Hemispheric Differences in the Acquisition of Descriptive Systems. *Brain and Language* 14: 144–173.

Goodwin, C., and Goodwin, M. H. (1992). Assessments and the Construction of Context. In A. Duranti and C. Goodwin (eds.), *Rethinking Context: Language as an Interactive Phenomenon*. Cambridge: Cambridge University Press.

Gray, K., and Holmes, S. (2020). Constraint in Emojis as Multimodal Public Pedagogy. *Computers and Composition* 55. https://doi.org/10.1016/j.compcom.2020.102552.

Greenhow, C., and Gleason, B. (2012). Twitteracy: Tweeting as a New Literary Practice. *The Educational Forum* 76: 464–478.

Grosz, P. G., Greenberg, G., De Leon, C., and Kaiser, E. (2023). A Semantics of Face Emoji in Discourse. *Linguistics and Philosophy* 46: 905–957. https://doi.org/10.1007/s10988-022-09369-8.

Group μ (1970). *A General Rhetoric*. Paris: Larousse.

Group μ (1992). *Traité du signe visuel: Pour une rhétorique de l'image*. Paris: Seuil.

Ha, J. F., and Longnecker, N. (2010). Doctor–Patient Communication: A Review. *The Ochsner Journal* 10(1): 38–43.

Haas, C., and Takayoshi, P. (2011). Young People's Everyday Literacies: The Language Features of Instant Messaging. *Research in the Teaching of English* 45(4): 378–404.

Haggard, E. A., and Isaacs, K. S. (1966). Micro-momentary Facial Expressions as Indicators of Ego Mechanisms in Psychotherapy. In L. A. Gottschalk and A. H. Auerbach (eds.), *Methods of Research in Psychotherapy*, 154–165. New York: Appleton-Century-Crofts.

Hall, E. T. (1959). *The Silent Language*. New York: Anchor.

Halliday, M. (1985). *Introduction to Functional Grammar*. London: Arnold.

Hand, C. J., Burd, K., Oliver, A., and Robus, C. M. (2020). Interactions between Text Content and Emoji Types Determine Perceptions of Both Messages and Senders. *Computers in Human Behavior Reports* 8. https://doi.org/10.1016/j.chbr.2022.100242.

Hariman, R., and Lucaites, J. L. (2011). *No Caption Needed: Iconic Photographs, Public Culture, and Liberal Democracy*. Chicago: University of Chicago Press.

Harper, C. (2022). Emojis Can Help You Communicate Quickly and Clearly. *Psychology Today*. www.psychologytoday.com/ca/blog/articles-heterodoxy/202207/emojis-can-help-you-communicate-quickly-and-clearly.

Harris, P. A., et al. (2019). The REDCap Consortium: Building an International Community of Software Platform Partners. *Journal of Biomedical Informatics* 95: 103208. https://doi.org/10.1016/j.jbi.2019.103208.

Hassel, H., and Phillips, C. (2022). *Materiality and Writing Studies: Aligning Labor, Scholarship, and Teaching*. Urbana, IL: National Council of Teachers of English.

He, S., Renne, A., Argandykov, D., Convissar, D., and Lee, J. (2022). Comparison of an Emoji-Based Visual Analog Scale with a Numeric Rating Scale for Pain Assessment. *Journal of the American Medical Association* 328(2): 208–209. https://doi.org/10.1001/jama.2022.7489.

Helprin, M. (2009). *Digital Barbarism: A Writer's Manifesto*. New York: Harper Collins.

Hickok, G., Bellugi, U., and Klima, E. S. (2001). Sign Language in the Brain. *Scientific American* 284(6): 58–65.

Hinsie, L. E., and Campbell, R. J. (1970). *Psychiatric Dictionary*. Oxford: Oxford University Press.

Hjortsjö, C.-H. (1970). *Man's Face and Mimic Language*. Lund: Studentlitteratur.

Hobbs, R. (2017). *Create to Learn: Introduction to Digital Literacy*. London: Wiley-Blackwell.

Hodges, C., Moore, S., Lockee, B., Trust, T., and Bond, A. (2020). The Difference Between Emergency Remote Teaching and Online Learning. *Educause Review*. https://er.educause.edu/articles/2020/3/the-difference-between-emergency-remote-teaching-and-online-learning.

Holton, D., and Symons, D. (2021). Emojis and Their Place in the Mathematics Classroom. *Australian Primary Mathematics Classroom* 26: 30–34.

Hsiao, C. (2010). Enhancing Children's Artistic and Creative Thinking and Drawing Performance through Appreciating Picture Books. *International Journal of Art & Design Education* 29(2): 143–152.

Hu, Y., Manikonda, L., and Kambhampati, S. (2014). What We Instagram: A First Analysis of Instagram Photo Content and User Types. In *Eighth International AAAI Conference on Weblogs and Social Media*, 595–598. AAAI Press.

Huckin, T. (1992). Context-Sensitive Text Analysis. In G. Kirsh and P. A. Sullivan (Eds.), *Methods and Methodology in Composition Research*, 84–104. Carbondale, IL: Southern Illinois University Press.

Huxley, A. (1942). *The Art of Seeing*. London: Harper & Brothers.

Jaeger, S. R., and Ares, G. (2017). Dominant Meanings of Facial Emoji: Insights from Chinese Consumers and Comparison with Meanings from Internet Resources. *Food and Quality Preference* 62: 275–283.

Jakobson, R. (1942). *Kindersprache, Aphasie und algemeine Lautgesetze*. Uppsala: Almqvist and Wiksell.

Jakobson, R. (1960). Linguistics and Poetics. In T. A. Sebeok (ed.), *Style and Language*, 34–45. Cambridge, MA: MIT Press.

Johnson, M. (1987). *The Body in the Mind: The Bodily Basis of Meaning, Imagination and Reason*. Chicago: University of Chicago Press.

Kalantzis, M., and Cope, B. (2012). *Literacies*. Cambridge: Cambridge University Press.

Kan, I. P., Alexander, M. P., and Verfaillie, M. (2009). Contribution of Prior Semantic Knowledge to New Episodic Learning in Amnesia. *Journal of Cognitive Neuroscience* 21: 938–944.

Kandola, A., Edwards, K., Muller, M., et al. (2023). Digitally Managing Depression: A Fully Remote Randomized Attention-Placebo Controlled Trial. medRxiv. https://doi.org/10.1101/2023.04.05.23288184.

Kaye, L. (2018). Why Psychology Needs to Start Taking Emoji Seriously. *The British Psychological Society*. www.bps.org.uk/blog/why-psychology-needs-start-taking-emoji-seriously.

Kendon, A. (1972). Some Relationships Between Body Motion and Speech: An Analysis of an Example. In R. Seigman and B. Pope Elmsford (eds.), *Studies in Dyadic Communication*, 68–99. New York: Pergamon Press.

Kharbach, M. (2022). Emojis in Learning. *Educational Technology and Mobile Learning*. www.educatorstechnology.com/2021/09/emojis-in-education-tools-and-apps-for.html.

Kiger, M. E, and Varpio, L. (2020). Thematic Analysis of Qualitative Data: AMEE Guide No. 131. *Medical Teacher* 42(8): 846–854.

Kim, M., Knotts, T. L., Albers, N. D., and James, K. E. (2022). Emoji Use as a Catalyst for Relationship Building and Sustaining Attention in Online Classes: An Empirical Study. *Educational Science* 12: 874. https://doi.org/10.3390/educsci12120874.

King, M. (2016). Using Emojis to Teach Critical Reading Skills. *Edutopia*. www.edutopia.org/article/using-emojis-to-teach-critical-reading-skills-marissa-king/.

Kirk, H., Vidgen, B., Röttger, P., and Hale, S. A. (2021). Hatemoji: A Test Suite and Adversarially-Generated Dataset for Benchmarking and Detecting Emoji-Based Hate. Oxford University Research Archive. https://ora.ox.ac.uk/objects/uuid:0570eaf5-e729-4ef5-b27a-b6d511abcdc3.

Kirley, E., and McMahon, M. (2018). The Emoji Factor: Humanizing the Emerging Law of Digital Speech. *Tennessee Law Review* 85(2): 1–61.

Klyukanov, I. E. (2005). *Principles of Intercultural Communication*. Boston, MA: Allyn and Bacon.

Korzybski, A. (1921). *Manhood of Humanity: The Science and Art of Human Engineering*. New York: E. P. Dutton & Company.

Korzybski, A. (1933). *Science and Sanity*. Brooklyn, NY: Institute of General Semantics.

Kress, G. (2003). *Literacy in the New Media Age*. New York: Routledge.

Kurniawan, F. (2016). The Use of Audiovisual Media in Teaching Speaking. *English Education Journal* 7: 180–193.

Lai, S., Lee, J., and He, S. (2021). Emoji for the Medical Community – Challenges and Opportunities. *JAMA Network* 326(9): 795–796. https://doi.org/10.1001/jama.2021.8409.

Lakoff, G. (1979). The Contemporary Theory of Metaphor. In A. Ortony (ed.), *Metaphor and Thought*, 220–251. Cambridge: Cambridge University Press.

Lakoff, G. (1987). *Women, Fire, and Dangerous Things: What Categories Reveal about the Mind*. Chicago: University of Chicago Press.

Lakoff, G., and Johnson, M. (1980). *Metaphors We Live By*. Chicago: Chicago University Press.

Lakoff, G., and Johnson, M. (1999). *Philosophy in Flesh: The Embodied Mind and Its Challenge to Western Thought*. New York: Basic.

Langacker, R. W. (1987). *Foundations of Cognitive Grammar*. Stanford, CA: Stanford University Press.

Langacker, R. W. (1990). *Concept, Image, and Symbol: The Cognitive Basis of Grammar*. Berlin: Mouton de Gruyter.

Langacker, R. W. (1999). *Grammar and Conceptualization*. Berlin: Mouton de Gruyter.

Langer, S. (1948). *Philosophy in a New Key*. Cambridge, MA: Harvard University Press.

Langer, S. K. (1937). *An Introduction to Symbolic Logic*. New South Wales: Allen and Unwin.

Langer, S. K. (1950). The Principles of Creation in Art. *Hudson Review* 2: 520–521.

Lea, M. R., and Street, B. V. (2006). The "Academic Literacies" Model: Theory and Applications. *Theory Into Practice* 45(4): 368–377.

Lebduska, L. (2014). Emoji, Emoji, What for Art Thou? *Harlot*. http://harlotofthearts.org/index.php/harlot/article/view/186/157.

Lee, A. C. K., Tang, S. W., Yu, G. K. K., and Cheung R. T. F. (2008). The Smiley as a Simple Screening Tool for Depression after Stroke: A Preliminary Study. *International Journal of Nursing Studies* 45(7): 1081–1089.

Lee, S. J., Back, A. L., Block, S. D., and Stewart, S. K. (2002). Enhancing Physician–Patient Communication. *Hematology* 2002(1): 464–483.

Lesniak, E., and Grzybowski (2021). The Role of Emoticons in the Comprehension of Emotional and Non-emotional Messages in Dyslexic Youth: A Preliminary Study. *Frontiers in Psychology* 12. https://doi.org/10.3389/fpsyg.2021.693287.

Levy, R. I. (1975). *Tahitians: Mind and Experience in the Society Islands*. Chicago: University of Chicago Press.

Li, L., Flynn, K., DeRosier, M., Weiser, G., and Austin-King, K. (2021). Social-Emotional Learning Amidst COVID-19 School Closures: Positive Findings from an Efficacy Study of Adventures Aboard the S.S. GRIN Program. *Frontiers in Education* 6. www.frontiersin.org/articles/10.3389/feduc.2021.683142/full.

Lin, T. S., and Luo, Y. (2023). Health Persuasion through Emoji: How Emoji Interacted with Information Source to Predict Health Behaviors in COVID-19 Situation. *Social*

Science and Medicine Population Health 21: 101343. https://doi.org/10.1016/j.ssmph.2023.101343.

Lindberg, S. (1994). New Farmers' Movements in India as Structural Response and Collective Identity Formation: The Cases of the Shetkari Sanghatana and the BKU. *The Journal of Peasant Studies* 21: 95–125.

Lindeberg, S. (1994). Apparent Absence of Cerebrocardiovascular Disease in Melanesians: Risk Factors and Nutritional Considerations: The Kitava Study. [Unpublished dissertation]. University of Lund.

Liu, M. (2023). Are You Really Smiling? Display Rules for Emojis and the Relationship Between Emotion Management and Psychological Well-Being. *Frontiers in Psychology* 14. https://doi.org/10.3389/fpsyg.2023.1035742.

Lobe, B., et al. (2020). Qualitative Data Collection in an Era of Social Distancing. *International Journal of Qualitative Methods* 19(2). https://doi.org/10.1177/1609406920937875.

Locke, J. (1690). *An Essay Concerning Humane Understanding*. Oxford: Clarendon Press.

Logi, L., and Zappavigna, M. (2021). A Social Semiotics Perspective on Emoji: How Emoji and Language Interact to Make Meaning in Digital Messages. *New Media & Society* 25(12): 3222–3246. https://journals.sagepub.com/doi/abs/10.1177/14614448211032965.

Losh, E. (2015). Teaching Urban Digital Literacy Outside Schools. *Connected Learning Alliance*. https://clalliance.org/blog/teaching-urban-digital-literacy-outside-schools-part-3/.

Lotfinejad, N., Assadi, R., Aelami, M. H., and Pittet, D. (2020). Emojis in Public Health and How They Might Be Used for Hand Hygiene and Infection Prevention and Control. *Antimicrobial Resistance & Infection Control* 9. https://doi.org/10.1186/s13756-020-0692-2.

Lotman, J. (1990). *The Universe of the Mind: A Semiotic Theory of Culture*. Bloomington: Indiana University Press.

Lu, X., Ai, W., Chen, Z., Cao, Y., and Mei, Q. (2022). Emojis Predict Dropouts of Remote Workers: An Empirical Study of Emoji Usage on GitHub. *PLoS One* 17(1): e0261262.

Lu, X., Ai, W., Liu, X., et al. (2016). Learning from the Ubiquitous Language. In *Proceedings of the 2016 ACM International Joint Conference on Pervasive and Ubiquitous Computing*, 770–780. New York: Association for Computing Machinery. https://doi.org/10.1145/2971648.2971724.

Luria, A. R. (1947). *Traumatic Aphasia*. The Hague: Mouton.

Ma, W., Liu, R., Wang, L., and Vosiughi, S. (2020). Multi-resolution Annotations for Emoji Prediction. *Proceedings of the 2020 Conference on Empirical Methods in Natural Language Processing*, 6684–6694. Association for Computational Linguistics

Malinowski, B. (1922). *Argonauts of the Western Pacific*. New York: Dutton.

Malinowski, B. (1923). The Problem of Meaning in Primitive Languages. In C. K. Ogden and I. A. Richards, *The Meaning of Meaning*, 296–336. London: Routledge.

Malykhina, E. (2014). Fact or Fiction?: Video Games are the Future of Education. *Scientific American*. www.scientificamerican.com/article/fact-or-fiction-video-games-are-the-future-of-education/.

Mapes, A. C., and Hea, A. C. K. (2018). Devices and Desires: A Complicated Narrative of Mobile Writing and Device-Driven Ecologies. In J. Alexander and J. Rhodes (eds.), *The Routledge Handbook of Digital Writing and Rhetoric*, 73–83. New York: Routledge.

Marchetti, N. (2015), Karkemish: New Discoveries in the Last Hittite Capital. *Current World Archaeology* 70: 18–24.

Marder, B., Houghton, D., Erz, A., Harris, L., and Javornik, A. (2020). Smile(y) – and Your Students Will Smile with You? The Effects of Emoticons on Impressions, Evaluations, and Behaviour in Staff-to-Student Communication. *Studies in Higher Education* 45: 2274–2286.

Marengo, D., Giannotta, F., and Settanni, M. (2017). Assessing Personality Using Emoji: An Exploratory Study. *Personality and Individual Differences* 112: 74–78.

Marengo, D., Settanni, M., and Giannotta, F. (2019). Development and Preliminary Validation of an Image-Based Instrument to Assess Depressive Symptoms. *Psychiatry Research* 279: 180–185.

Markus, R. A. (1957). St. Augustine on Signs. *Phronesis* 2: 60–83.

Martinez, R. (2022). Should Clinicians Use Emojis When They Communicate with Each Other? *Stat.* www.statnews.com/2022/05/04/should-clinicians-use-emojis-when-communicating-with-each-other/.

Marzouk, S., He, S., and Lee, J. (2022). Emoji Education: How Students Can Help Increase Health Awareness by Making Emojis. *Journal of Medical Internet Research.* 8(4): e39059. https://doi.org/10.2196/39059.

Matsumoto, D. (1992). More Evidence for the Universality of a Contempt Expression. *Motivation and Emotion* 16: 363–368.

Matulewska, A., and Gwiazdowicz, D. J. (2020). Cyberbullying in Poland: A Case Study of Aggressive Messages with Emojis Targeted at the Community of Hunters in Urbanized Society. *Social Semiotics* 30: 379–395.

McCaffrey, T., and Matthews, P. G. (2017). An Emoji is Worth a Thousand Variables. *The Mathematics Teacher* 111(2): 96–102.

McCrea, S. M., and Robinson, T. P. (2011). Visual Puzzles, Figure Weights, and Cancellation: Some Preliminary Hypotheses on the Functional and Neural Substrates of These Three New WAIS-IV Subtests. *International Scholarly Research Notices.* https://doi.org/10.5402/2011/123173.

McDonald, K. (2007). Teaching L2 Vocabulary through Logic Puzzles. *Estudios de Lingüística Inglesa Aplicada* 7: 149–163.

McDonough, K., and Trofimovich, P. (2008) *Using Priming Methods in Second Language Research.* New York: Routledge.

McLuhan, M. (1960). Classrooms without Walls. In Edmund Carpenter (ed.), *Explorations in Communication*, 23–34. Boston, MA: Beacon Press.

McLuhan, M. (1962). *The Gutenberg Galaxy: The Making of Typographic Man.* Toronto: University of Toronto Press.

McLuhan, M. (1964). *Understanding Media: The Extensions of Man.* Cambridge, MA: MIT Press.

McLuhan, M. (1969). *Through the Vanishing Point.* New York: Harper & Row.

McLuhan, M. (1987). *Letters of Marshall McLuhan.* M. Molinaro and C. McLuhan (eds.). Oxford: Oxford University Press.

McLuhan, M., and Leonard, G. (1967). The Future of Education: The Class of 1989. *Look*, February 21, 23–24.

McNeill, D. (1992). *Hand and Mind: What Gestures Reveal about Thought.* Chicago: University of Chicago Press.

McNeill, D. (2005). *Gesture & Thought.* Chicago: University of Chicago Press.

Miller, H., Thebault-Spieker, J., Chang, S., et al. (2016). "Blissfully Happy" or "Ready to Fight": Varying Interpretations of Emoji. Association for the Advancement of Artificial Intelligence. www-users.cse.umn.edu/~bhecht/publications/ICWSM2016_emoji.pdf.

Mills, K. A., Stone, B. G., and Unsworth, L. (2020). Multimodal Aspects of Attitude. *Written Communication* 37: 074108831989797.

Moffitt, R. L., Padgett, C., and Grieve, R. (2021). The Impact of Emoji Use and Feedback Medium on Perceptions of Marker Personality in Online Assessment Feedback. *Learning and Individual Differences* 92. https://doi.org/10.1016/j.lindif.2021.102093.

Montoya, S. (2018). Defining Literacy. UNESCO, Institute for Statistics. https://gaml.uis.unesco.org/wp-content/uploads/sites/2/2018/12/4.6.1_07_4.6-defining-literacy.pdf.

Moore, C. A. (2017). Emoji as Visual Literacy. *Medium*. https://catherineannemoore.medium.com/emoji-as-visual-literacy-cbebe37cb99c.

Morris, C. W. (1938). *Foundations of the Theory of Signs*. Chicago: University of Chicago Press.

Morris, C. W. (1946). *Signs, Language and Behavior*. Englewood Cliffs, NJ: Prentice-Hall.

Moyer, P. S., Bolyard, J. J., and Spikell, M. A. (2002). What Are Virtual Manipulatives? *Teaching Children Mathematics* 8: 372–377.

Myers, V., and Colturi, J. (2022). Use of Emoji in the Health Care Setting: Helpful or Harmful? *Op-Med*. https://opmed.doximity.com/articles/use-of-emoji-in-the-health-care-setting-helpful-or-harmful.

Najda, N. (2016). Aphasic to Aphasic Interaction. In M. Danesi and S. Greco (eds.), *Case Studies in Discourse Analysis*, 46–57. Munich: Lincom Europa.

Neuman, Y., Danesi, M., and Vilenchik, D. (2023). *Using AI for Dialoguing with Texts: From Psychology to Cinema and Literature*. New York: Routledge.

Novak, P., Smailović, J., Sluban, B., and Mozetič, I. (2015). Sentiment of Emojis. *PLoS ONE* 10(12): e0144296. https://doi.org/10.1371/journal.pone.0144296.

Nusrat, F., and Huang, Y. (2021). Less Talking, More Empathy: How to Use Emojis to Help People Feel Good. *Association of Marketing Theory and Practice Proceedings*. https://digitalcommons.georgiasouthern.edu/amtp-proceedings_2021/21.

O'Reilly-Shah, V., Lynde, G., and Jabaley, C. (2018). Is It Time to Start Using the Emoji in Biomedical Literature? *British Medical Journal* 363: k5033. https://doi.org/10.1136/bmj.k5033.

Oakley, T., and Pascual, E. (2017). Conceptual Blending Theory. In B. Dancygier (ed.), *The Cambridge Handbook of Cognitive Linguistics*, 423–448. Cambridge: Cambridge University Press.

Obler, L. K., and Gjerlow, K. (1999). *Language and the Brain*. Cambridge: Cambridge University Press.

Ogden, C. K. (1932). *Opposition: A Linguistic and Psychological Analysis*. London: Paul, Trench, and Trubner.

Olson, D. (1977). *Media and Symbols: The Forms of Expression, Communication and Education*. Chicago: University of Chicago Press.

Ong, W. (1982). *Orality and Literacy*. New York: Methuen.

Paggio, P., and Tse, A. Ping Ping (2022). Are Emoji Processed Like Words? An Eye-Tracking Study. *Cognitive Science* 46(2). https://doi.org/10.1111/cogs.13099.

Peirce, C. S. (1931–1958). *Collected Papers of Charles Sanders Peirce*, vols. 1–8. C. Hartshorne and P. Weiss (eds.). Cambridge, MA: Harvard University Press.

Pereira-Kohatsu, J., Quijano-Sánchez, L., Liberatore, F., and Camacho-Collados, M. (2019). Detecting and Monitoring Hate Speech in Twitter. *Sensors* 19: 4654.

Perryman-Clark, S., Kirkland, D. E., Jackson, A., and Smitherman, G. (2015). *Students' Right to Their Own Language: A Critical Sourcebook*. Boston, MA: St Martin's.

Petcoff, O. W. (2022a). *Q1 traditional writing most frequently used words*. Voyant tools. https://voyant-tools.org/?corpus=c4a48bece58a1384950623e03577e86f&palette=d3_cat10&view=Summary.

Petcoff, O. W. (2022b). *Q1 traditional writing word cloud*. Voyant tools. https://voyant-tools.org/?corpus=c4a48bece58a1384950623e03577e86f&palette=d3_cat10&whiteList=&view=Cirrus.

Petcoff, O. (2023). Exploring Emoji as a Semioliteracy Instructional Tool in the Developmental Reading and Writing Classroom. [Unpublished doctoral dissertation]. Texas Tech University. https://ttu-ir.tdl.org/items/d318792c-b00d-463e-ba32-f02d795fc0d3.

Petrilli, S. (2009). *Signifying and Understanding: Reading the Works of Victoria Lady Welby and the Significs Movement*. Berlin: Mouton de Gruyter.

Piaget, J. (1969). *The Child's Conception of the World*. Totowa: Littlefield, Adams and Company.

Piriyatamwong, P. (2022). Emojional Intelligence: 😳 How AI Can Predict Your Next Emoji. *The AI Journal*. https://aijourn.com/emojional-intelligence-😳-how-ai-can-predict-your-next-emoji/.

Rankin, L. (2013). *Mind over Medicine: Scientific Proof That You Can Heal Yourself*. Carlsbad, CA: Hay House.

Rasula, S., Bukhsh, Q., and Batool, S. (2011). A Study to Analyze the Effectiveness of Audio Visual Aids in Teaching Learning Process at University Level. *Procedia: Social and Behavioral Sciences* 28: 78–81.

Rathore, A. S. (2022). Emojis for What Words Can't Say. *Dailyexcelsior.com*, December 18.

Reddy, M. J. (1979). The Conduit Metaphor: A Case of Frame Conflict in Our Language about Language. In A. Ortony (ed.), *Metaphor and Thought*, 284–310. Cambridge: Cambridge University Press.

Renne, A., He, S., and Lee, J. (2022). An Emoji-Based Visual Analog Scale Compared with a Numeric Rating Scale for Pain Assessment. *JAMA* 328(19): 1980–1981.

Riad, R. Allodi, M. W., Siljehag, E., et al. (2021). How I Feel About My School: Adaptation and Validation of an Educational Well-Being Measure among Young Children in Sweden. *International Journal of Environmental Research in Public Health* 18(10). https://doi.org/10.3390/ijerph18105075.

Riordan, M. (2017). The Communicative Role of Non-Face Emojis: Affect and Disambiguation. *Computers in Human Behavior* 76: 75–86.

Robson, R. (2019). Emoji Law 101. https://robsonlaw.com/2019/11/emoji-law-101/.

Rong, S., Wang, W., Mannan, U. A., et al. (2022). An Empirical Study of Emoji Use in Software Development Communication. *Information and Software Technology* 148(6). http://doi.org/10.1016/j.infsof.2022.106912.

Rosenblatt, L. (2005). *Making Meaning with Texts: Selected Essays*. Portsmouth, NH: Heinemann.

Saldaña, J. (2020). *The Coding Manual for Qualitative Researchers*. London: Sage.

San-Martin, M., Delgado-Bolton, R., and Vivanco, L. (2017). Role of a Semiotics-Based Curriculum in Empathy Enhancement: A Longitudinal Study in Three Dominican Medical Schools. *Frontiers in Psychology* 8. https://doi.org/10.3389/fpsyg.2017.02018.

Saussure, F. de (1916). *Cours de linguistique générale*. Paris: Payot.

Savage, B. M., Lujan, H. L., Thipparthi, R. R., and DiCarlo, S. E. (2017). Humor, Laughter, Learning, and Health! A Brief Review. *Advances in Physiology Education* 41(3): 341–347.

Scheffler, T., Brandt, L., Fuente, M., and Nenchev, I. (2021). The Processing of Emoji-Word Substitutions: A Self-Paced-Reading Study. *Computers in Human Behavior* 127. https://doi.org/10.1016/j.chb.2021.107076.

Schmandt-Besserat, D. (1978). The Earliest Precursor of Writing. *Scientific American* 238: 50–59.

Schmandt-Besserat, D. (1992). *Before Writing*, 2 vols. Austin: University of Texas Press.

Seargeant, P. (2019). *The Emoji Revolution: How Technology Is Shaping the Future of Communication*. Cambridge: Cambridge University Press.

Searle, J. R. (1969). *Speech Acts: An Essay in the Philosophy of Language*. Cambridge: Cambridge University Press.

Searle, J. R. (1976). A Classification of Illocutionary Acts. *Language in Society* 5: 1–23.

Selfe, C. L. (2017). *Multimodal Composition: Resources for Teachers*. Columbia, SC: Hampton Press.

Semetsky, I., and Stables, A. (2014). *Pedagogy and Edusemiotics: Theoretical Challenges/Practical Opportunities*. Rotterdam: Sense Publishers.

Semetsky, I. R. (2019). *Semiotic Subjectivity in Education and Counseling: Learning with the Unconscious*. London: Routledge.

Sexton, W., and Beegle, R. (2020). Academic Language in an Emoji World. *A Journal of the Texas Council of Teachers of English Language Arts* 50(2): 6–10.

Shafer, G. (1998). Whole Language: Origins and Practice. *Language Arts Journal of Michigan* 14: 18–21.

Sharma, K. (2023). Can Emojis Improve Doctor–Patient Communication? *HealthSite*. www.thehealthsite.com/author/kashish-sharma/.

Shipka, J. (2011). *Toward a Composition Made Whole*. Pittsburgh, PA: University of Pittsburgh Press.

Siegel R. M., Anneken, A., Duffy, C., et al. (2015). Emoticon Use Increases Plain Milk and Vegetable Purchase in a School Cafeteria without Adversely Affecting Total Milk Purchase. *Clinical Therapeutics* 37(9): 1938–1943.

Singh, A., and Husain, Z. (2020). The Use of Emoticons in Text-Based Therapy. *International Journal of Creative Research Thoughts* 8(9): 3860–3866. https://ijcrt.org/papers/IJCRT2009492.pdf.

Skemp, R. R. (1971). *The Psychology of Learning Mathematics*. Harmondsworth: Penguin.

Sketchley, M. (2022). Emojis in the English Classroom. *ELT Experiences*. https://eltexperiences.com/emojis-in-the-english-classroom/.

Skiba, D. J. (2016). Face with Tears of Joy Is Word of the Year: Are Emoji a Sign of Things to Come in Health Care? *Nursing Education Perspectives* 37: 56–57.

Smith, L. R., and Sanderson, J. (2015). I'm Going to Instagram It! An Analysis of Athlete Self-Presentation on Instagram. *Journal of Broadcasting & Electronic Media* 59: 342–358.

Sonnevend, J. (2020). A Virus as an Icon: The 2020 Pandemic in Images. *American Journal of Cultural Sociology* 8: 451–461.

Sontag, S. (1978). *Illness as Metaphor*. New York: Farrar, Straus & Giroux.

Stavans, A., Eden, M. T., and Azar, L. (2021). Multilingual Literacy: The Use of Emojis in Written Communication. In E. O. Breuer, E. Lindgren, and A. Stavans (eds.), *Multilingual Literacy*: 82–99. Bristol: Multilingual Matters.

Street, B. (2003). What's "New" in New Literacy Studies? Critical Approaches to Literacy in Theory and Practice. *Current Issues in Comparative Education* 5(2): 77–91.

Stewart, M. A. (1995). Effective Physician–Patient Communication and Health Outcomes: A Review. *Canadian Medical Association Journal* 152(9): 1423–1433.

Stonbraker S., Porras T., and Schnall R. (2020). Patient Preferences for Visualization of Longitudinal Patient-Reported Outcomes Data. *Journal of the American Medical Information Association* 27(2): 212–224.

Stough, C., Roberts, J., and Downey, L. A. (2011). Workplace Culture Emotional Intelligence and Trust in the Prediction of Workplace Outcomes. *International Journal of Business Science and Applied Management* 6(1): 30–40.

Street, B. (2013). Literacy in Theory and Practice: Challenges and Debates over 50 Years. *Theory into Practice* 52(1): 52–62.

Street, B. K. (2003). What's "New" in New Literacy Studies? Critical Approaches to Literacy in Theory and Practice. *Current Issues in Comparative Education* 5(2): 77–91.

Suleiman, H., and Eltom, E. (2019). Using Emoji to Improve Female Students' Coherence in Writing at Qassim University. *Advances in Language and Literary Studies* 10(4): 57–62. http://doi.org/10.7575/aiac.alls.v.10n.4p.57.

Szeto, M. D., Barber, C., Ranpariya, V. K., et al. (2022). Emojis and Emoticons in Health Care and Dermatology Communication: Narrative Review. *Journal of Medical Internet Reach Dermatology* 5(3): e33851. https://doi.org/10.2196/33851.

Tannen, D. (1989). *Talking Voices*. Cambridge: Cambridge University Press.

Taylor, J. S. H., Davis, M. H., and Rastle, K. (2017). Comparing and Validating Methods of Reading Instruction Using Behavioural and Neural Findings in an Artificial Orthography. *Journal of Experimental Psychology* 146: 826–858.

Teixera, M. I. (2022). Can Emojis Help You Learn a Language? *Lingoda*. https://blog.lingoda.com/en/can-emojis-help-you-learn-a-language/.

Tham, J. C. K. (2018). Interactivity in an Age of Immersive Media: Seven Dimensions for Wearable Technology, Internet of Things, and Technical Communication. *Technical Communication* 65(1): 46–65.

Thomas, J. J., and Cook, K. A. (2005). *Illuminating the Path: The R&D Agenda for Visual Analytics*. National Visualization and Analytics Center.

Thompson, C. A., Novotny, P. J., Bartz, A., Yost, K. J., and Sloan, J. A. (2018). Development of Novel Emoji Scale to Measure Patient-Reported Outcomes in Cancer Patients. *Journal of Clinical Oncology* 36(7). https://ascopubs.org/doi/10.1200/JCO.2018.36.7_suppl.174.

Tolman, E. (1932). *Purposive Behavior in Animals and Men*. New York: Appleton-Century-Crofts.

Tulving, E. (1972). Episodic and Semantic Memory. In E. Tulving and W. Donaldson (eds.), *Organization of Memory*, 23–46. New York: Academic.

Tuohy, P. (2018). Reading Graphic Medicine. *Journal of the Medical Library Association* 106(3): 387–390.

Van Dam, L., Rietstra, S., Van der Drift, E., et al. (2019). Can an Emoji a Day Keep the Doctor Away? An Explorative Mixed-Methods Feasibility Study to Develop a Self-Help App for Youth with Mental Health Problems. *Frontiers in Psychiatry* 23. https://doi.org/10.3389/fpsyt.2019.00593.

Vance, E. (2010). Augustine (Aurelius Augustinus), Bishop of Hippo (354–430). In T. A. Sebeok and M. Danesi (eds.), *Encyclopedic Dictionary of Semiotics*, 65–67. Berlin: Mouton de Gruyter.

Vareberg, K. R., Vogt, O., and Berndt, M. (2022). Putting Your Best Face Forward: How Instructor Emoji Use Influences Students' Impressions of Credibility, Immediacy, and Liking. *Education Information Technology* 28: 6075–6092. https://doi.org/10.1007/s10639-022-11421-w.

Vespoor, M. H. (2008). Cognitive Linguistics and Its Applications to Second Language Teaching. In N. H. Hornberger (ed.), *Encyclopedia of Language and Education*, 23–36. Boston, MA: Springer.

Vygotsky, L. S. (1961). *Thought and Language*. Cambridge, MA: MIT Press.

Wagner, A., Marusek, S., and Yu, W. (2020). Sarcasm, the Smiling Poop, and e-Discourse Aggressiveness: Getting Far Too Emotional with Emojis. *Social Semiotics* 30: 305–311.

Wagner, A., and Yu, W. (2021). Machiavellian Apparatus of Cyberbullying: Its Triggers Igniting Fury with Legal Impacts. *International Journal of the Semiotics of Law* 34: 945–963. https://doi.org/10.1007/s11196-021-09841-x.

Weigle, S., and Caprino, K. (2018). Tips for Using Emojis and Bitmoji in the Literacy Classroom. *Literacy Now*. www.literacyworldwide.org/blog/literacy-now/2018/09/27/tips-for-using-emojis-and-bitmoji-in-the-literacy-classroom.

Weise, H., and Labrenz, A. (2021). Emoji as Graphic Discourse Markers: Functional and Positional Associations in German Whatsapp® Messages. In D. van Olmen and J. Šinkūnienė (eds.), *Pragmatic Markers and Clause Peripheries*, 277–300. Amsterdam: John Benjamins.

Weissman, B., and Tanner, D. (2018). A Strong Wink between Verbal and Emoji-Based Irony: How the Brain Processes Ironic Emojis During Language Comprehension. *PLoS One* 13(8): e0201727. https://doi.org/10.1371/journal.pone.0201727.

Weiß M., Gutzeit J., Rodrigues J., Mussel P., and Hewig J. (2019). Do Emojis Influence Social Interactions? Neural and Behavioral Responses to Affective Emojis in Bargaining Situations. *Psychophysiology* 56(4): e13321. https://doi.org/10.1111/psyp.13321.

Welby, V. (1897). *Grains of Sense*. London: J. M. Dent.

Willoughby J. F., and Liu, S. (2018). Do Pictures Help Tell the Story? An Experimental Test of Narrative and Emojis in a Health Text Message Intervention. *Computers in Human Behavior* 79: 75–82.

Wiseman, S., and Gould, S. J. J. (2018). Repurposing Emoji for Personalised Communication: Why 🍕 Means "I Love You." In *Proceedings of the 2018 CHI Conference on Human Factors in Computing Systems*, 21–26. Association for Computing Machinery. http://doi.org/10.1145/3173574.3173726.

Wood, E., Zivcakova, L., Gentile, P., et al. (2012). Examining the Impact of Off-Task Multi-tasking with Technology on Real-Time Classroom Learning. *Computers & Education* 58(1): 365–374.

Wood, I., and Ruder, S. (2016). Emoji as Emotion Tags for Tweets. *Emotion and Sentiment Analysis Workshop.* LREC 2016.

Yakin, V., and Eru, O. (2017). An Application to Determine the Efficacy of Emoji Use on Social Marketing Ads. *International Journal of Social Sciences and Education Research* 3(1): 230–240.

Yang, X., and Liu, M. (2021). The Pragmatics of Text-Emoji Co-occurrences on Chinese Social Media. *Pragmatics* 31(1): 144–172.

Yenawine, P. (1997). Thoughts on Visual Literacy. In J. Flood, S. Brice Heath, and D. Lapp (eds.), *Handbook of Research on Teaching Literacy through the Communicative and Visual Arts*, 845–847. New York: Routledge.

Yokoi, T., and Jordan, J. (2022). Using Emojis to Connect with Your Team. *Harvard Business Review*. https://hbr.org/2022/05/using-emojis-to-connect-with-your-team.

Yuasa, M., Saito, K., and Mukawa, N. (2011). Brain Activity When Reading Sentences and Emoticons: An fMRI Study of Verbal and Nonverbal Communication. *Electronics and Communication in Japan* 94(5): 17–24.

Zhou, S., and Landa, N. (2021). Using Emoticons to Reduce Transactional Distance: Navigating the Contextual Complexities of COVID-19 Imposed Virtual Learning Spaces. *Paper Presented at the Fifteenth General Conference: The Future of African Higher Education.*

Zipf, G. K. (1935). *The Psycho–Biology of Language: An Introduction to Dynamic Philology*. Boston, MA: Houghton–Mifflin.

Zipf, G. K. (1949). *Human Behavior and the Principle of Least Effort*. Boston, MA: Addison–Wesley

Index

Printed in the USA
CPSIA information can be obtained
at www.ICGtesting.com
CBHW071331010624
9426CB00003B/40